An Innovative Design of

BIPOLAR PROSTHESIS

(THE BHU HIP DEVICE)

Prof. A.K Rai

Co author

Dr. Abhijeet Kunwar

Dr. Shubhanshu Shekhar

Dr. Anand Saurabh

BlueRose ONE.com

Stories Matter

NewDelhi • London

BLUEROSE PUBLISHERS
India | U.K.

BlueRose ONE.com
Stories Matter
NewDelhi • London

For permissions requests or inquiries regarding this publication, please contact:

BLUEROSE PUBLISHERS
www.BlueRoseONE.com
info@bluerosepublishers.com
+91 8882 898 898
+4407342408967

ISBN: 978-93-5741-246-9

Cover design: Aman Sharma

First Edition: September 2023

When the Religion was Strong and Science Weak
Man Mistook Magic for Medicine

Now that Science is Strong and Religion Weak,
Man Mistakes Medicine for Magic

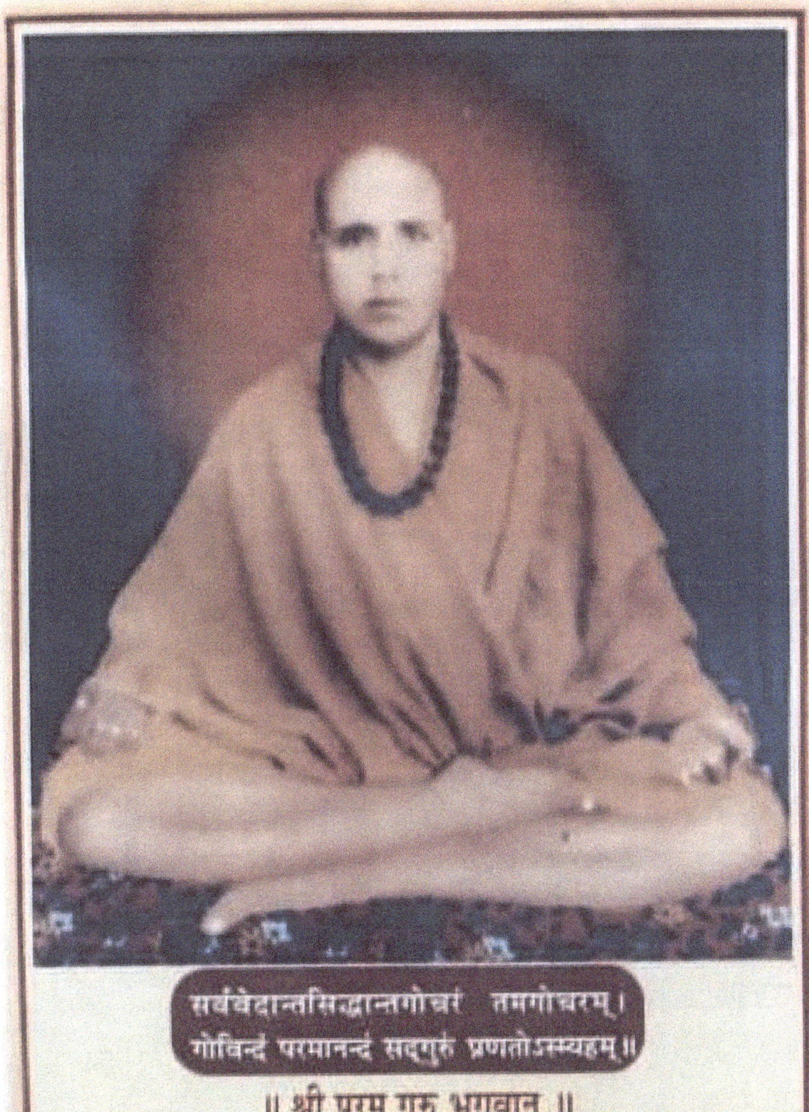

Swami Param Gyanananda Ji Maharaj Paramhans

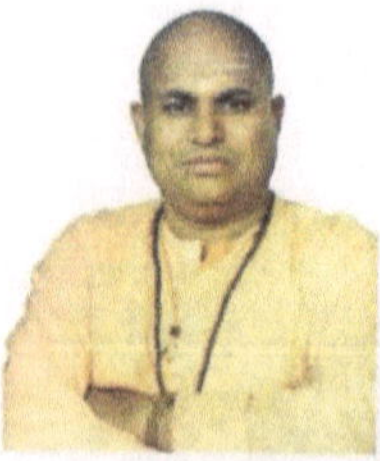

काशी हिन्दू विश्वविद्यालय के आयुर्विज्ञान संस्थान के डा0 अनिल कुमार राय अस्थिरोग विभाग के भूतपूर्व चिकित्सक एवं आचार्य रहे हैं। अपने विषय में इनकी कार्य कुशलता सर्वज्ञात है। देश विदेश से निराश लौटे हुए अनेक रोगियों को भी इन्होने आरोग्य दान देकर उनके जीवन में खुशियॉ उकेरी हैं। अपने विदेश प्रवास के दौरान इन्होने कूल्हे के प्रत्यारोपण के लिए जो उपकरण (Device) इजाद किये हैं उसने तो अपने क्षेत्र में मानो धूम मचा दी है। खासकर पूर्वांचल तथा बिहार के गरीब रोगियों के लिए यह उपकरण वरदान सिद्ध हुआ है क्योंकि विदेश से आयतित Device की तुलना में डाक्टर राय द्वारा प्रदत्त उपकरण काफी सस्ता तो है ही अपेक्षाकृत अधिक सुविधाजनक भी है। देश विदेश के अधिकांश चिकित्सक इस बाईपोलर प्रोस्थेसिस का इस्तेमाल कर रहे हैं। यह Device डा0 साहब के कुशल बौद्धिक क्षमता का परिचायक है।

डा0 राय से मेरा परिचय अत्यन्त पुराना है कोई चार दशकों से भी अधिक। ये शुरू से ही अपने छात्र जीवन में अत्यधिक मेधावी तथा कुशाग्रबुद्धि सम्पन्न रहे हैं। इनसे मेरा सम्बन्ध गुरू घर के नाते है। अपनी सफलता एवं अनुभवशीलता के पीछे ये एकमात्र श्रेय अपने आध्यात्मिक गुरू श्रीमत् परमहंस स्वामी परम ज्ञानानन्द जी महाराज को देते हैं। शरू में ही इनके सिद्ध गुरूदेव ने इन्हें जीनियस होने का आशीर्वाद दिया था। डा0 राय उसके सचमुच अनुरूप हैं। सन् 2000 ई0 में न्यूयार्क (अमेरिका) में आयोजित विश्व धर्म सम्मेलन में डाक्टर साहब मेरे साथ थे और वे वहाँ अपना वक्तृत्व भी दिया था। अंग्रेजी और हिन्दी दोनों भाषाओं मे इनकी वक्तृत्व प्रतिभा का तो कोई जोड़ ही नहीं। निबन्ध लेखन कार्य में इनकी भाषा की अभिव्यक्ति देखकर पाठक पूछ पड़ते हैं कि ये डाक्टर अनिल चिकित्सक है अथवा भाषा में पी0एचडी0!

हृदय की उदारता, दयालुता, परोपकारिता और व्यवहार में पारदर्शिता तथा अभिमान शून्यता आदि गुणों के कारण इन्हें 'साधु' कहा जाय तो कुछ कम नहीं। इनकी सहृदयता के कायल समाज में असंख्य लोग हैं जिनकी इन्होने चिकित्सा के अलावा अन्य रूपों में भी बढ चढ़ कर मदद की है।

बहुमुखी प्रतिभा के धनी एक सुमानव के रूप में प्रख्यात डा0 अनिल राय अपनी चिकित्सीय कार्यक्षमता से आजन्म लोकसेवा करते रहे, इनकी कार्यकुशलता उत्तरोत्तर प्रखर से प्रखतर होती रहे ताकि जन सामान्य का अशेष उपकार इनसे हो ऐसा मैं आशुतोष भगवान विश्वनाथ एवं अपने परम गुरूदेव से बारम्बार कर जोड़कर विनती करते हुए अपने साधु ह्दय से अपनी हार्दिक शुभाशंसा व्यक्त करता हूँ।

स्वामी पूर्णानन्द पुरी,
रॉची झारखण्ड

FOREWARD

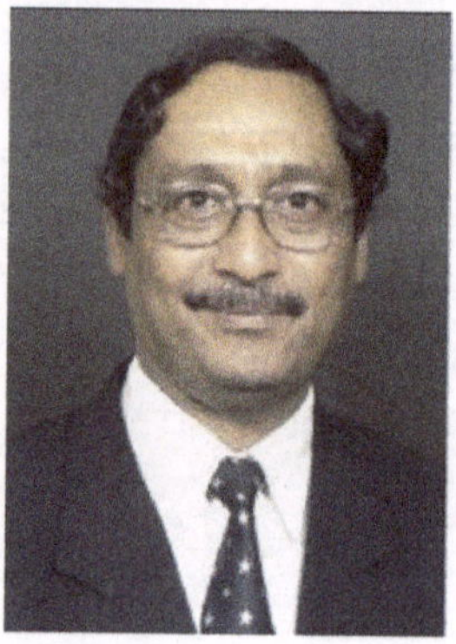

Prof Anil Kumar Rai has been my colleague in the department for more than three decades. After a vast experience in Hip Replacement Surgery in U K, when he returned India to join the department, his obsession was to develop a much economical option for hip replacement as he observed a high cost of THR implants not affordable by vast majority of Indians. He took this as his mission and started working on the project of modifying the existing bipolar available with an objective of providing results as good as THR and at the same time at much economical cost. For decades, he kept visiting metallurgic, Bio medical, Mechanical engineering departments and meeting doyens in the field of orthopaedic with continuously modifying and refining the model. He has compiled his thoughts and experiences while working on it in this book eloquently. The illustrations are easy to understand with several clinical photographs. His passion and hard work is apparent in various chapters written in a very simple language.

The book can be recommended to all who love the specialty of Orthopaedics with an eye on innovation.

Dr. S K SARAF MS, MNAMS, FICS
Ex. Professor and Head
Department of Orthopaedics
Institute of Medical Sciences
Banaras Hindu University, Varanasi

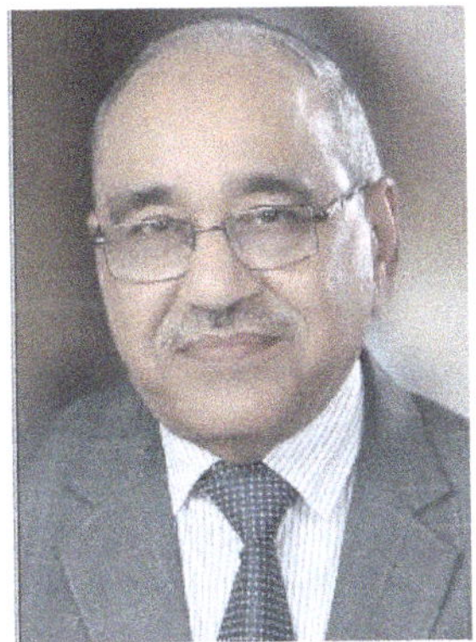
Prof. S.C. Goel 1979 - 2016

Replacement arthroplasty has been in vogue for a long time now. Modern orthopaedic surgery has changed radically. There is need of a cheap suitable alternative to total hip arthroplasty for Indian society. The prosthesis should permit movements of the hip to allow squatting and sitting cross legged and retain the movements for longer period as the problems of the sub-continent are different from western world.

Dr Anil Kumar Rai has developed a new bipolar prosthesis for the replacement of head of the femur in cases of fracture of neck of the femur. He has been a dedicated teacher for more than 23 years and has tried to put his experience in this book. He has described the biomechanics of hip and bipolar prosthesis and problem in design in detail. He has also dealt with preoperative problems and methods to solve them.

The language is easy format is readable and pleasant. Illustrations are well drawn.

Dr SC Goel
MS, FAMS, FASIF, FIGOF, FICS, Girdlestone Scholar (Oxon)
Professor and Head, Dept of Orthopaedics
Heritage Institute of Medical Sciences, Varanasi
Ex- Professor and Head, Department of Orthopedics, IMS
Banaras Hindu University, Varanasi, India
Past President, Trauma Society of India
Past President, Indian Orthopaedic Association

PREFACE

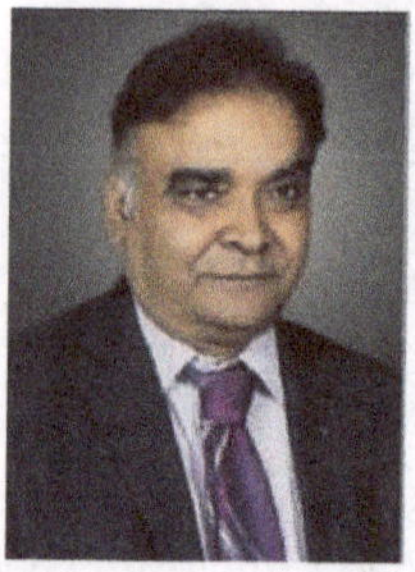

Prosthetic replacement for the hip Pathology is an unsolved quest, since many workers in the past found that the hemi replacement is not functioning up to the mark and the THR is not always a solution.

This book Is an extract of experience of the author working on and with this bipolar prosthesis for past 30 years.

This book is an answer for all those intellects managing hip Pathology who once in a while get stuck with the scenario of unsalvageable head in not so old patient where THR is always an overdo and results of bipolar does not encourage them to go head with it. It is actually an attempt to put the evolution of a bipolar prosthesis and the performance it has delivered on pages inform of this book via the patients who has been the part of this journey.

We agree that this is not a conventional orthopaedic handbook but actually is the passion of the author to develop something that fits to the society of low socioeconomic status yet not deprive them of any day to day activity.

This book is the result of work of brilliant minds of medical Sciences and mechanical engineering coming together to design something that could be a solution to the problems never answered before.

Chapter like "mathematical calculation" might appear little out of place in context of the topic but it is this basic thing that laid the foundation around which everything has revolved during design of this prosthesis.

Chapter on history of hip replacement is interesting in itself as it tells what surgeons in the past have done to get a pain less functional hip , how all those trials which now appears ridiculous actually paved the path for evolution of hip replacement in the form we see it now.

Designer changes once an orthopaedician goes through this topic he/she will be amazed to see that how little changes (put in place after great efforts and trials though) made in the design can greatly enhance the performance of the bipolar prosthesis.

Chapter on surgical approach is full of justifiable modifications to conventional approach described in literatures to make it easier and to achieve maximum benefit out of it.

Prof VK Shukla (Rector, Banaras Hindu University) and Prof. Anand Mohan (Dept. Electrical engineering IIT BHU) deserves a special vote of thanks as they bestowed their endless support and motivation from beginning of this journey.We are also thankful to Prof Tyagi (then workshop incharge, IIT,BHU) and Mr. Lalajee Vishwakarma (IIT,BHU,Workshop) who extended their helping hands when the foundation stones for this dream were laid.

This page will be incomplete until we mention how much we are thankful to Department of Forensic Medicine for providing us cadavers as and when needed.

CONTRIBUTORS

Prof (retd) A Bhattacharya
Department of mechanical engineering
IIT BHU

Dr. Manjaree Mishra
Associate Professor (Anesthesia)
Trauma Centre, IMS BHU

Dr Anand Saurabh
MBBS,MS (ortho)
Senior resident(ortho)
Trauma Centre IMS,BHU

&

Dr Shubhanshu Shekhar
MBBS MS(ortho)
Senior resident(ortho)
Trauma centre IMS BHU

ACKNOWLEDGEMENT

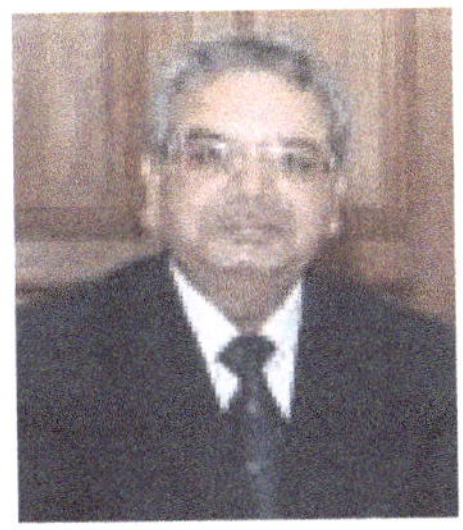

Prof. Anil Kumar Rai is well known to me since last two decades as an outstanding faculty and surgeon of Department of Orthopaedics, Institute of Medical Sciences, Banaras Hindu University, Varanasi-221005, India. Through my personal interactions, I observed that Prof. Raihas obtained state–of-the–art training in orthopaedic surgery from UK that makes him distinctly different from many others.

I am extremely happy to mention that Prof. Rai developed an innovative model of hip device that is extremely cost effective. He has successfully implanted this hip device in patients; demonstrating and validating its professional feasibility.

It is my greatest pleasure to learn that Prof. Rai has compiled his professional accomplishments on 'hip device' for its publication. I believe, this would be quite useful to the professionals in the field.

(Anand Mohan)
Former Director, NIT Kurukshetra, Haryana
Former Member, Executive Council, BHU, Varanasi
Former Vice-Chairman, Board of Governors, IIT- BHU, Varanasi
Former Chairman, ASE Panel under ARMREB, DRDO, Ministry of Defence, Govt. of India, New Delhi
Former Head, Department of Electronics Engineering, IT-BHU

CONTENTS

THE HIP JOINT

The hip is a true ball-and-socket joint surrounded by powerful and well-balanced muscles, enabling a wide range of motion in several physical planes while also exhibiting remarkable stability. As the structural link between the lower extremities and the axial skeleton, the hips not only transmit forces from the ground up but also carry forces from the trunk, head and neck, and upper extremities. It meets the four characteristics of a synovial or diarthrodial joint: it has a joint cavity; joint surfaces are covered with articular cartilage; it has a synovial membrane producing synovial fluid, and; it is surrounded by a ligamentous capsule.

The cup-shaped acetabulum is formed by the innominate bone with contributions from the ilium (approximately 40% of the acetabulum), ischium (40%) and the pubis (20%). In the skeletally immature these three bones are separated by the triradiate cartilage – fusion of this starts to occur around the age of 14 – 16 years and is complete usually by the age of 23.

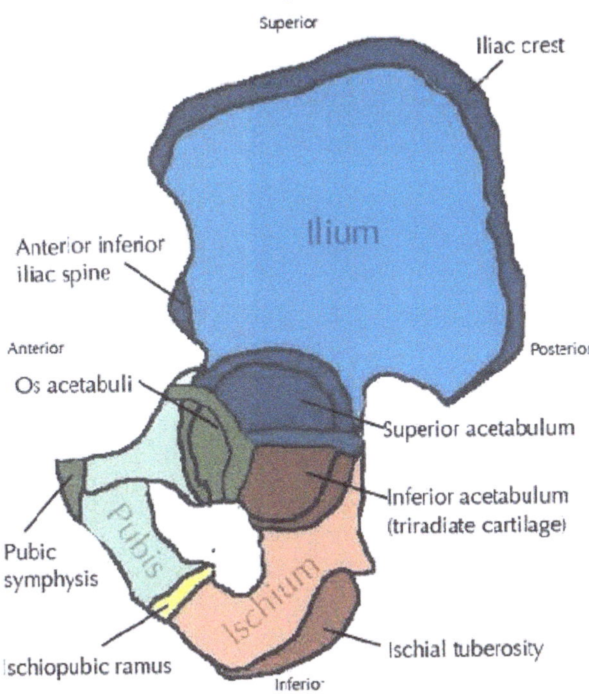

Ossification of the femur begins in the 7th fetal week. In early childhood, only a single proximal femoral physis exists. During the first year of life, the medial portion of this physis grows faster than the lateral, creating an elongated femoral neck by 1 year of age. The capital femoral epiphysis begins to ossify at approximately 4 months in girls and 5 to 6 months in boys. The ossification center of the trochanteric apophysis appears at 4 years in boys and girls. The proximal femoral physis is responsible for the metaphyseal growth in the femoral neck, whereas the trochanteric apophysis contributes to the appositional growth of the greater trochanter and less to the metaphyseal growth of the femur. Fusion of the proximal femoral and trochanteric physes occurs at about the age of 14 in girls and 16 in boys.

The socket of the hip is completed by the inferior transverse ligament. Attached to the rim of the acetabulum is the fibrocartilaginous labrum. Although it makes less of a contribution to joint stability than the glenoid labrum in the shoulder it does serve its purpose. It plays a role in normal joint development and in distribution of forces around the joint. It has also been suggested it plays a role in restricting movement of synovial fluid to the peripheral compartment of the hip, thus helping exert a negative pressure effect within the hip joint.

The labrum runs around the circumference of the acetabulum terminating inferiorly where the transverse acetabular ligament crosses the inferior aspect of the acetabular fossa. It attaches to the bony rim of the acetabulum and is quite separate from the insertion of the capsule.

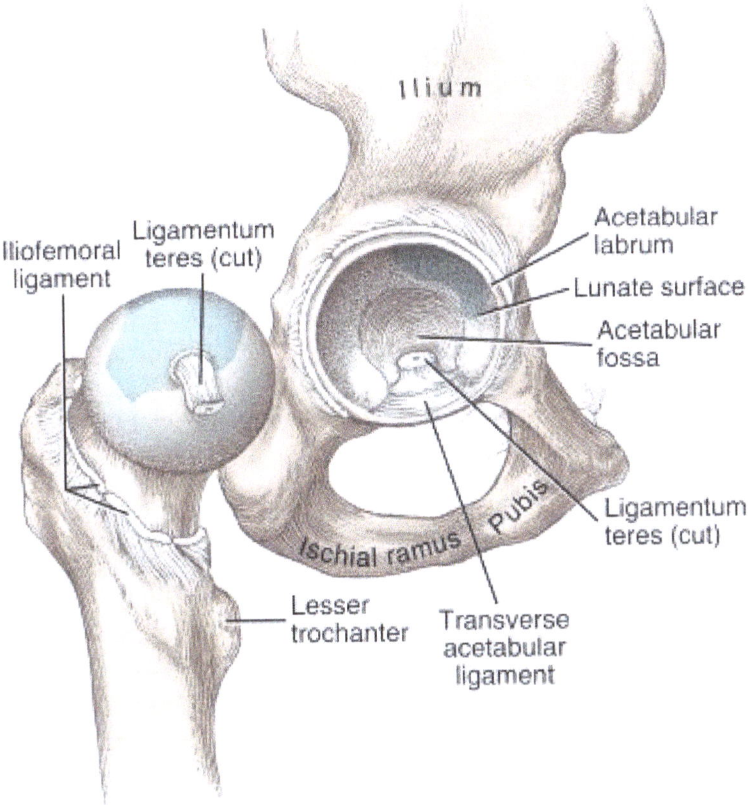

The labrum receives a vascular supply from the obturator and the superior and inferior gluteal arteries. These ascend in the reflected synovial layer on the capsule and enter the peripheral aspect of the labrum. It has been observed that labral tears are most likely to occur at the junction of labrum and articular cartilage - this area has been termed the 'watershed region'.

The femoral head is covered with a corresponding articular cartilage beyond the reaches of the acetabular brim to accommodate the full range of motion. The covered region forms approximately 60 to 70% of a sphere. There is an uncovered area on the central area of the femoral head – the fovea capitis – for the femoral insertion of the ligamentum teres. The ligamentum teres, while containing a blood supply does not contribute to the stability of the joint. It is covered in synovium, so while it is intra-articular it is actually extra-synovial.

Angulation of femur

There are two angulations made by the head and neck of the femur in relation to the shaft **1.Angle of torsion** occurs in the transverse plane between an axis through the femoral head and neck and an axis through the distal femoral condyles (version of neck) **2.Angle of inclination** occurs in the frontal plane between an axis through the femoral head and neck and the longitudinal axis of the femoral shaft (neck shaft angle).

The head of the femur is attached to the femoral shaft by the femoral neck, which varies in length depending on body size. The neck-shaft angle is usually 125±5° in the normal adult. Coxa valga being the condition when this value exceeds 130° and Coxa vara when the inclination is less than 120°. The importance of this feature is that the femoral shaft is laterally displaced from the pelvis, thus facilitating freedom for joint motion. If there is significant deviation in angle outside this typical range, the lever arms used to produce motion by the abductor muscles will either be too small or too large.

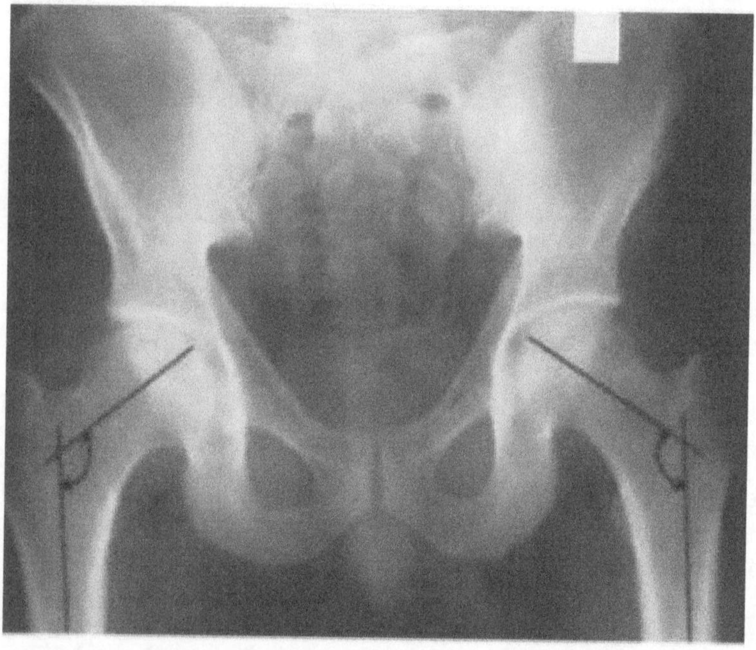

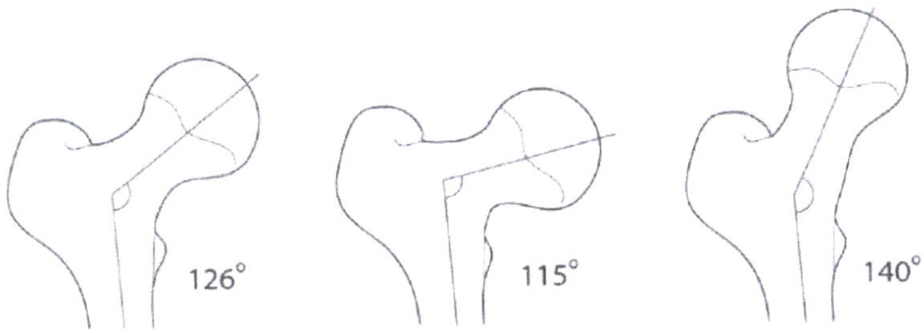

Normal	Coxavar	Coxa valga

The neck-shaft angle steadily decreases from 150° after birth to 125° in the adult due to remodelling of bone in response to changing stress patterns.

The femoral neck in the average person is also rotated slightly anterior to the coronal plane, this anterior inclination of head and neck with respect to shaft of femur is called antiversion and varies between 15-20 degree.

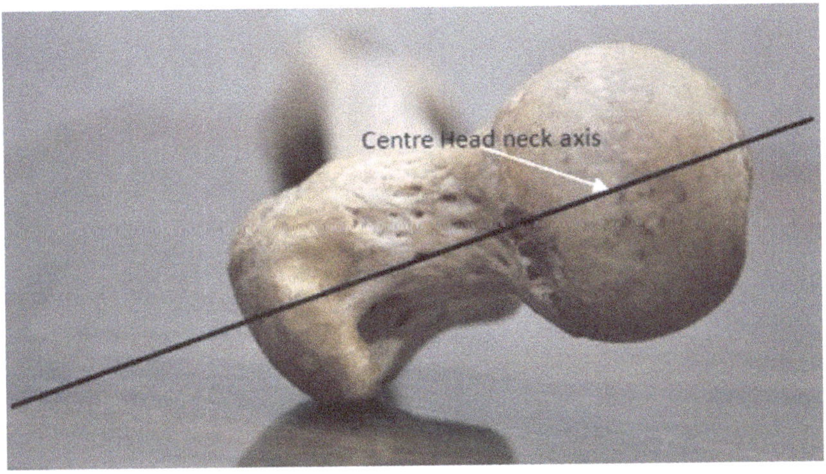

LIGAMENTS AND CAPSULAR ANATOMY

The joint capsule is strong. While the ball and deep socket configuration naturally gives the hip great stability the ligamentous capsule undoubtedly contributes significantly. The capsule is formed by an intertwining of three separate entities. The iliofemoral ligament can be seen anterior to the hip in the form of an inverted 'Y'. It spans, in a spiralling fashion, from its proximal attachment to the ilium to insert along the intertrochanteric line. It is taught inextension and relaxed in flexion keeping the pelvis from tilting posteriorly in upright stance and limiting adduction of the extended lower limb. It is the strongest ligament in the body. Inferior and posterior to the iliofemoral ligament, and blending into its medial edge, the pubofemoral ligament contributes to the strength of the anteroinferior portion of the capsule. This is perhaps the weakest of the four ligaments. Posteriorly the ischiofemoral ligament completes the main ligamentous constraints – from it ischial attachment medially it inserts laterally on superolateral aspect of the femoral neck, medial to the base of the greater trochanter.

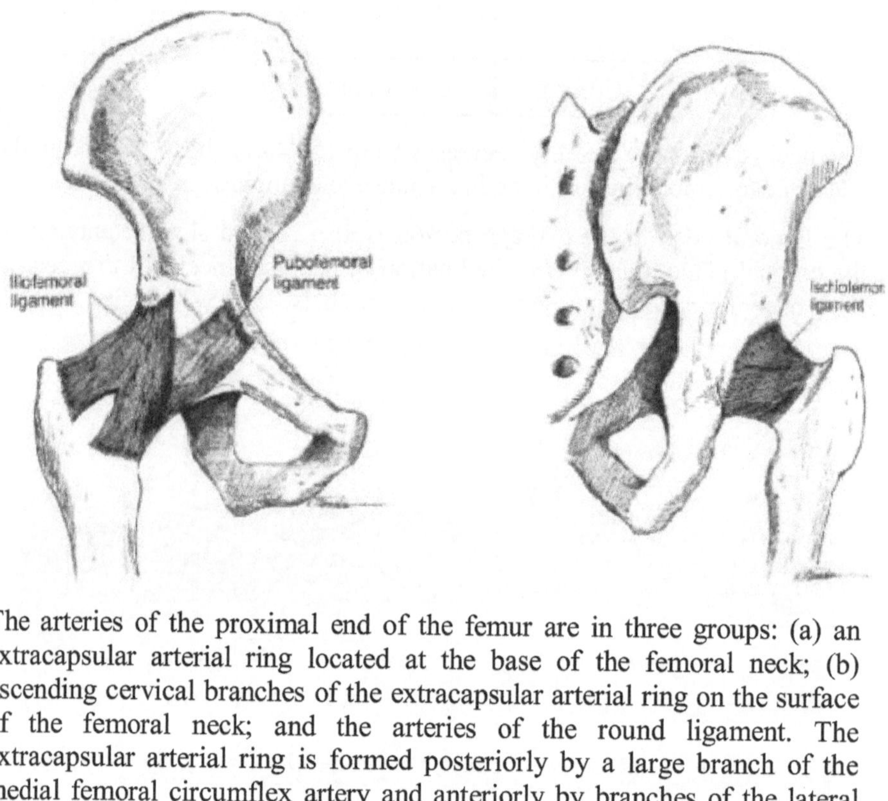

The arteries of the proximal end of the femur are in three groups: (a) an extracapsular arterial ring located at the base of the femoral neck; (b) ascending cervical branches of the extracapsular arterial ring on the surface of the femoral neck; and the arteries of the round ligament. The extracapsular arterial ring is formed posteriorly by a large branch of the medial femoral circumflex artery and anteriorly by branches of the lateral femoral circumflex artery. The superior and inferior gluteal arteries also have minor contributions to this ring. The ascending cervical branches arise from the extracapsular arterial ring. Anteriorly they penetrate the capsule of the hip joint at the intertrochanteric line and posteriorly, they pass beneath the orbicular fibers of the capsule. The ascending cervical branches pass upward under the synovial reflections and fibrous prolongations of the femoral head from its neck. These arteries are known as retinacular arteries, described initially by Weitbrecht. The proximity of the retinacular arteries to bone puts them at risk for injury in any fracture of the femoral neck. As the ascending cervical arteries traverse the superficial surface of the femoral neck, they send many small branches into the metaphysis of the femoral neck. Additional blood supply to the metaphysis arises from the extracapsular arterial ring and may include anastomoses with intramedullary branches of the superior nutrient artery system, branches of the ascending cervical arteries, and the subsynovial intra-articular ring. This excellent vascular supply to the metaphysis explains the absence of avascular changes in the femoral neck as opposed to the head. The ascending cervical arteries can be divided into four groups (anterior, medial, posterior, and lateral) based on their relationship to the femoral neck. Of these four, the lateral group provides most of the blood supply to the femoral head and neck. At the margin of the articular cartilage on the surface of the neck of the femur, these vessels form a second ring, which Chung has termed the subsynovial intra-articular arterial ring. At the subsynovial intra-articular ring, epiphyseal arterial branches arise that enter the femoral head. Once the arteries from the subsynovial intra-articular ring penetrate the femoral head, they are termed the epiphyseal arteries.

The artery of the ligamentum teres is a branch of the obturator or the medial femoral circumflex artery. The functional presence of this artery has been variably reported in the literature. Howe et al found that although the vessels of the ligamentum teres did supply vascularity to the femoral head, they were often inadequate to assume the major nourishment of the femoral head after a displaced femoral neck fracture.

Thus the vascular supply to the femoral head has three sources as noted (a) a small vessel found within the ligamentum teres (present in about 80% of the population), (b) a supply from the medullary canal and (c) an anastamosis of vessels creeping around the femoral neck. Where the last group of vessel being most significant in supplying blood to head, and the artery in ligamentum teres (foveal artery) being least significant and contributes to only 20 % of total circulation .

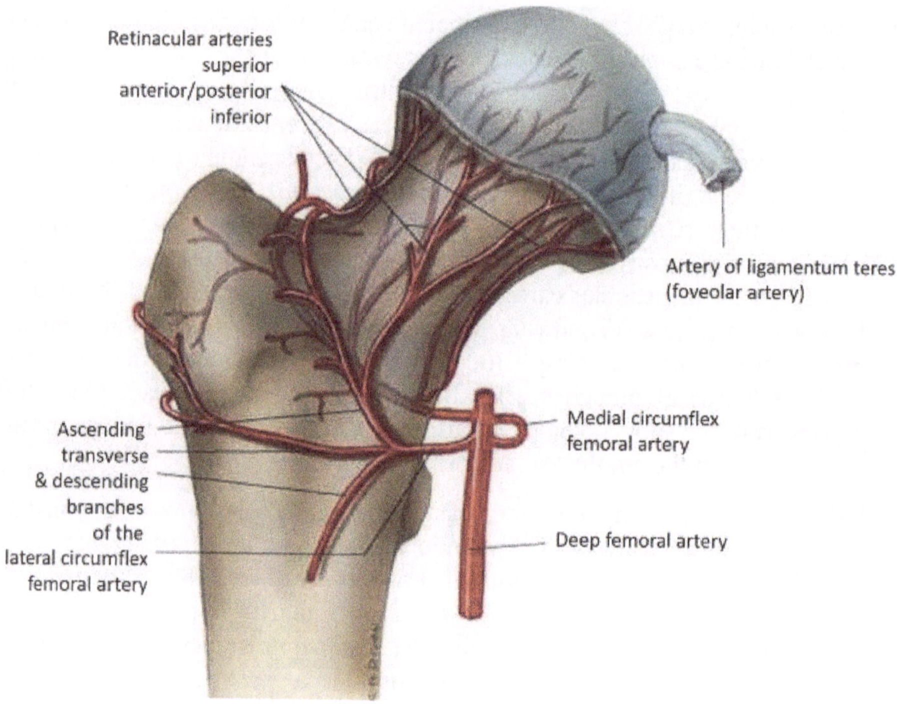

MUSCULAR ANATOMY

The 22 muscles acting on the hip joint not only contribute to stability but also provide the forces required for movement of the hip. The musculature of the hip and thigh is invested in a fibrous layer the fascia lata. This is a continuous fibrous sheath surrounding the thigh. Proximally it is attached to the inguinal ligament, lip of the iliac crest, posterior aspect of the sacrum, the ischial tuberosity, the body of the pubis and the pubic tubercle. Its inelasticity functions to limit bulging of the thigh muscles thus improving the efficiency of their contractions.

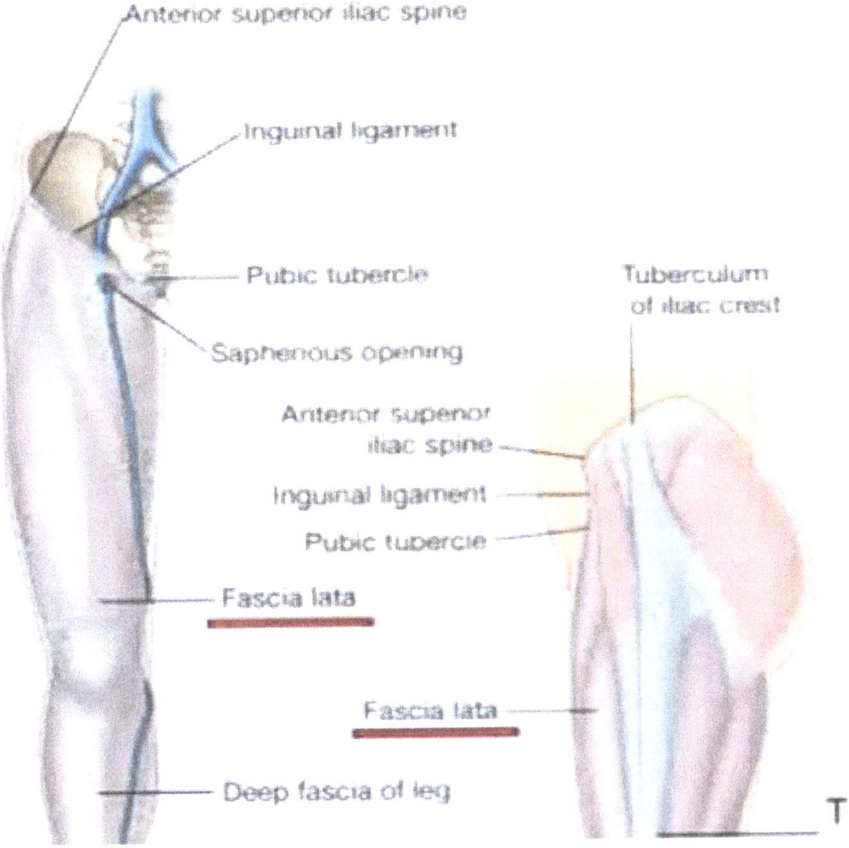

The major flexor of the hip joint is iliopsoas. This comprises psoas major and minor, and iliacus. Psoas major arises from T12-L5 vertebral bodies and insets into the lesser trochanter. It is joined at the level of the inguinal ligament to form the iliopsoas Iliopsoas is the most powerful hip flexor but it is also aided by sartorius, rectus femoris and tensor fascia latae (TFL). **Sartorius**, innervated by the femoral nerve, runs from ASIS to insert medial to the tibial tuberosity. It also contributes to abduction and external rotation. Rectus femoris also arises from the ASIS and inserts into the tibial tuberosity by way of the patella ligament.

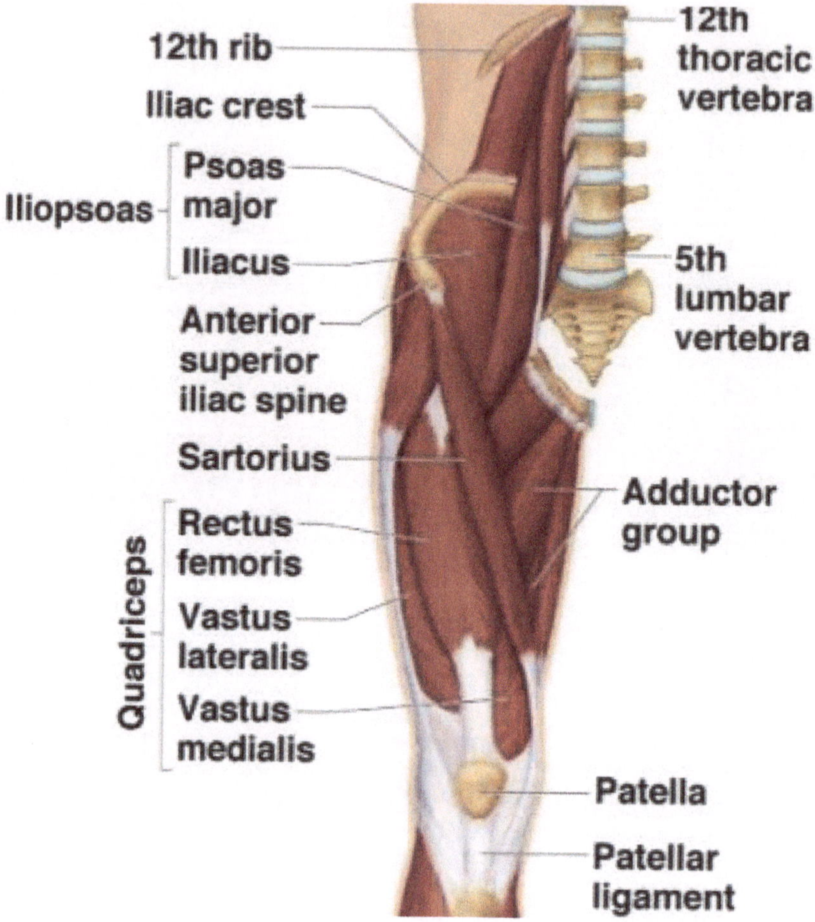

The largest and most powerful extensor of the hip is gluteus maximus. It is also the most superficial. Running from the lateral aspect of the dorsal sacral surface, posterior part of the ilium and thoracolumbar fascia it inserts into the iliotibial tract and gluteal tuberosity on the femur.

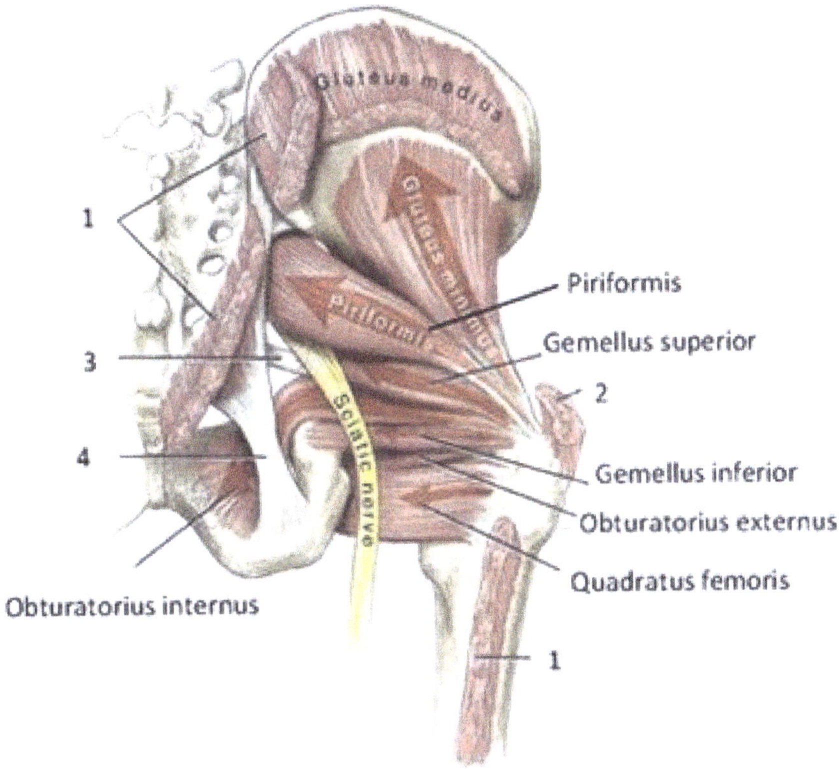
Gluteus medius
Gluteus minimus
Piriformis
Sciatic nerve
1
Piriformis
Gemellus superior
3
2
4
Gemellus inferior
Obturatorius externus
Quadratus femoris
Obturatorius internus
1

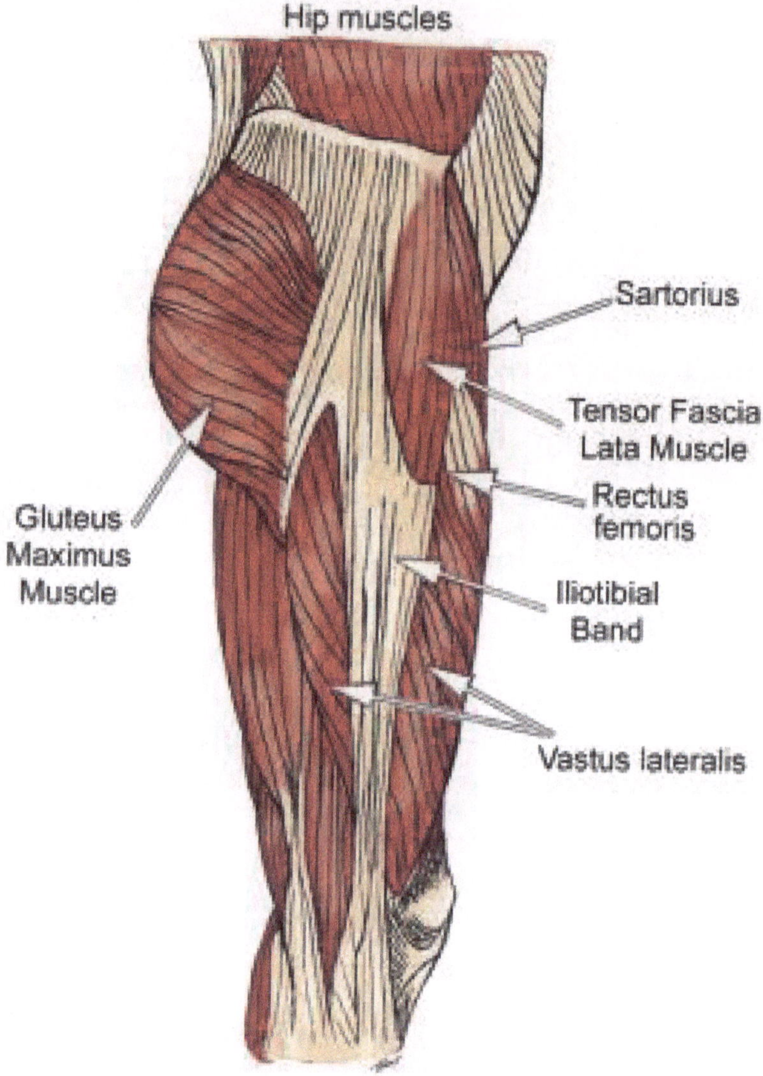

The principal abductors include gluteus medius and minimus. Lying beneath the fascia lata, the proximal insertion of gluteus medius into the iliac crest is almost continuous with it. From its broad based proximal attachment it appears like an upside-down triangle inserting into a relatively narrow base on the lateral aspect of the greater trochanter. Gluteus minimus is deep again to gluteus medius arsing proximally from the gluteal surface of the ilium and inserting deep to the gluteus medius on the anterolateral aspect of the greater trochanter - both gluteus medius and minimus are innervated by the superior gluteal nerve.

Piriformis runs laterally from the pelvic surface of the sacrum to the apex of the greater trochanter of the femur. It also contributes to external rotation and extension of the hip. Posteriorly, inferior to the piriformis, are the short external rotators all running in a horizontal fashion. From superior to inferior, these consist of the superior gemelli, obturator internus, inferior gemelli, and quadratus femoris. All play a role in external rotation and adduction of the hip and all receive branches from L5-S1 in the sacral plexus.

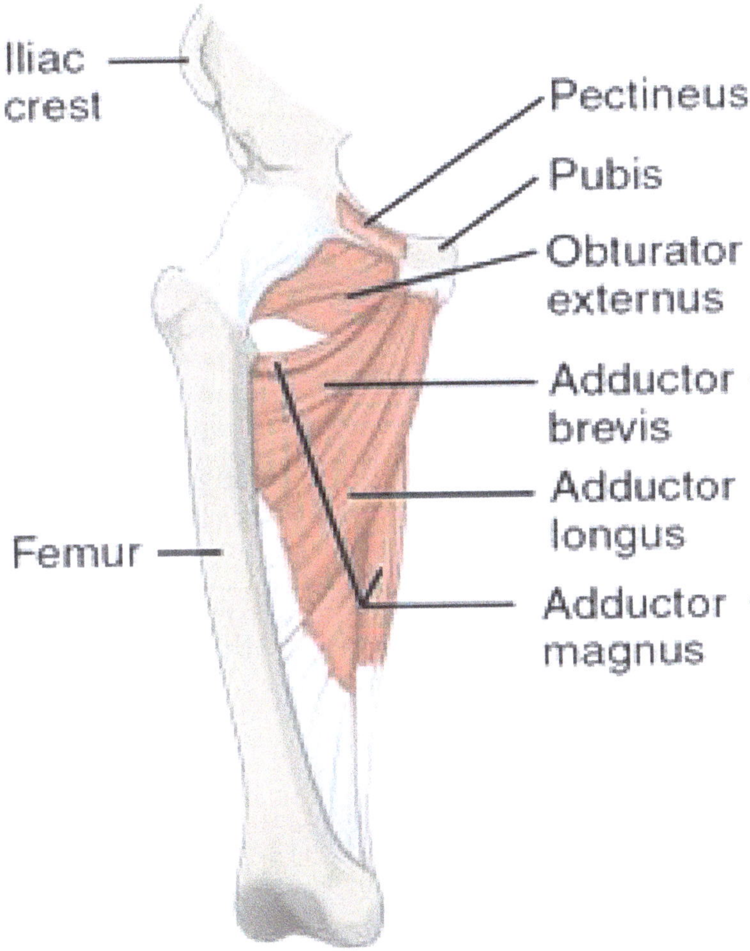

Hip adductors include the obturator externus arising from the outer surface of the obturator membrane and inserting into the trochanteric fossa. Pectineus attaches at the pectin pubis and inserts into the femur along the pectineal line and linea aspera. It also contributes to external rotation and some flexion. Adductor longus attaches medial to pectineus on the superior pubic ramus and inserts distally to the pectineus along the middle third of the linea aspera – it contributes to hip flexion up to 70°. Adductor brevis arises from the inferior pubic ramus and inserts proximal to adductor longus into the proximal one third of the linea aspera. Adductor magnus arises from the inferior pubic rami, ischial ramus and ischial tuberosity. It inserts distally into the medial lip of the linea aspera but also has a more tendinous insertion into the medial condyle of the femur. It contributes also to extension and external rotation. Adductor minimus runs from the inferior pubic ramus into the medial lip of the linea aspera also contributing to external rotation. Gracilis is the only adductor that inserts distal to the knee joint. It arises inferior to the pubic ramus below the pubis symphysis. All the adductors receive an innervation from the obturator nerve.

BIOMECHANICS OF THE HIP

The static loading of the hip joint has been frequently approximated with a simplified, two-dimensional analysis performed in the frontal plane. When the weight of the body is being borne on both legs, the centre of gravity is centred between the two hips and its force is exerted equally on both hips. Under these loading conditions, the weight of the body minus the weight of both legs is supported equally on the femoral heads, and the resultant vectors are vertical.

In a single leg stance, the effective centre of gravity moves distally and away from the supporting leg since the nonsupporting leg is now calculated as part of the body mass acting upon the weight-bearing hip. This downward force exerts a turning motion around the centre of the femoral head – the moment is created by the body weight, and its moment arm,(distance from femur to the centre of gravity). The muscles that resist this movement are offset by the combined abductor muscles. This group of muscles includes the upper fibres of the gluteus maximus, the tensor fascia lata, the gluteus medius and minimus, and the piriformis and obturator internus. The force of the abductor muscles also creates a moment around the centre of the femoral head; however this moment arm is considerably shorter than the effective lever arm of body weight. Therefore the combined force of the abductors must be a multiple of body weight.

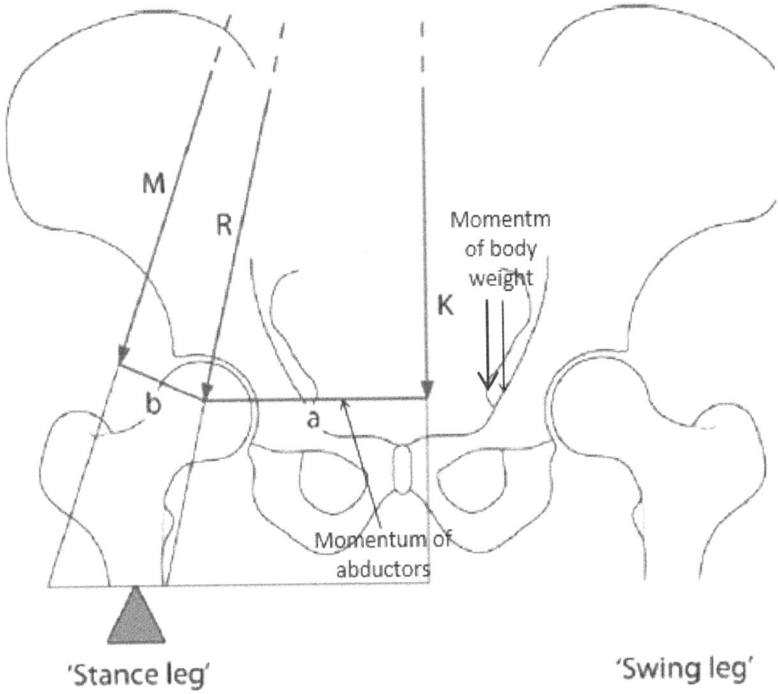

The magnitude of the forces depends critically on the lever arm ratio, which is that ratio between the body weight moment arm and the abductor muscle moment arm. Typical levels for single leg stance are three times bodyweight, corresponding to a level ratio of 2.5. Thus, anything that increases the lever arm ratio also increases the abductor muscle force required for gait and consequently the force on the head of the femur as well.

Management of painful hip disorders aim to reduce the joint reaction force. Bearing in mind the basic principles outlined above, this can be achieved by reducing the body weight or its moment arm, or helping the abductor force or its moment arm. Increases in body weight will have a particularly harmful effect on the total compressive forces applied to the joint. The effective loading of the joint can be significantly reduced by bringing the centre of gravity closer to the centre of the femoral head. This can be accomplished by limping, however the lateral movements required take a considerable amount of energy and is a much less efficient means of ambulation. Another strategy to reduce joint reaction force involves using a cane or walking stick in the opposite hand. The two-dimensional static analysis indicates that the joint reaction force can be reduced by 50% when approximately 15% body weight is applied to the cane. The substantial reduction in the joint reaction force, predicted when a cane is used for support arises because the cane-ground reaction force acts at a much larger distance from the centre of the hip than the abductor muscles. Thus, even when a relatively small load is applied to the cane, the contribution it makes to the moment opposing body weight is large enough to significantly decrease the demand placed on the abductor muscles. Hence sharing some of the hip load to shoulders through cane.

REFERENCES

1. Damien P. Byrne*, Kevin J. Mulhall and Joseph F. Baker Anatomy & Biomechanics of the Hip *The Open Sports Medicine Journal,* 2010; *4;* 51-57

2. Campbell JD, Higgs R, Wright K, Leaver-Dunn D. Pevis, hip and thigh injuries. In: Schenck RC, Guskiewicz KM, Holmes CF, Eds. Athletic Training and Sports Medicine. Rosemount: American Academy of Orthopaedic Surgeons 2001; p. 399.

3. Mosca VS. Pitfalls in diagnosis: the hip. Pediatr Ann 1989; 18(1): 12-4, 16-8, 23.

4. McCarthy J, Barsoum W, Puri L, *et al.* The role of hip arthroscopy in the elite athlete. Clin Orthop Relat Res 2003; (406): 71-4.

5. Philippon M, Schenker M, Briggs K, Kuppersmith D. Femoroacetabular impingement in 45 professional athletes: associated pathologies and return to sport following arthroscopic decompression. Knee Surg Sports Traumatol Arthrosc 2007; 15(7): 908-14.

6. Byrd J. Gross anatomy. In: Byrd J, Ed. Operative Hip Arthroscopy, 2nd ed. New York: Springer Science + Business Media, Inc. 2004; pp. 100-9.

7. Schuenke M, Schulte E, Schumacher U. THIEME Atlas of Anatomy. In: Ross L, Lamperti E, Eds. General Anatomy of the Musculoskeletal System. New York: Thieme New York 2006.

8. Moore K, Ed. Clinically Oriented Anatomy. 3rded. Baltimore: Williams and Wilkins 1992.

9. Byrd JWT. Indications and contraindications. In: Byrd JWT, Ed. Operative Hip Arthroscopy. 2nd ed. New York: Springer Science Business Media, Inc. 2005. Kim YH. Acetabular dysplasia and osteoarthritis developed by an eversion of the acetabular labrum. Clin Orthop Relat Res 1987; (215): 289-95.

10. Tanabe H. Aging process of the acetabular labrum--an electronmicroscopic study. Nippon Seikeigeka Gakkai Zasshi 1991; 65(1): 18-25.

11. Ferguson SJ, Bryant JT, Ganz R, Ito K. An *in vitro* investigation of the acetabular labral seal in hip joint mechanics. J Biomech 2003; 36(2): 171-8.

12. Seldes RM, Tan V, Hunt J, *et al.* Anatomy, histologic features, and vascularity of the adult acetabular labrum. Clin Orthop Relat Res 2001; (382): 232-40.

13. McCarthy JC, Noble PC, Schuck MR, *et al.* The Otto E. Aufranc Award: the role of labral lesions to development of early degenerative hip disease. Clin Orthop Relat Res 2001; (393): 25-37.

14. Gray AJ, Villar RN. The ligamentum teres of the hip: an arthroscopic classification of its pathology. Arthroscopy 1997; 13(5): 575-8.

15. Birnbaum K, Prescher A, Hessler S, Heller KD. The sensory innervation of the hip joint--an anatomical study. Surg Radiol Anat 1997; 19(6): 371.

FRACTURE NECK FEMUR

Hip fractures have a bimodal age distribution: Approximately 97% occur in patients over 50 years of age (the incidence increases with age), and only 3% in patients under 50. In the latter group, they occur most commonly between 20 and 40 years of age, usually in men, and are due to high-energy trauma associated with sports and industrial and motor-vehicle accidents. In this young group, most hip fractures are subtrochanteric or basicervical. In contrast, fractures of the hip in patients between 40 and 50 years of age usually occur in alcoholics or patients with multiple medical diseases, whose fractures are related to osteoporosis.

Femoral neck fractures and intertrochanteric fractures occur with about the same frequency. Nearly nine of 10 hip fractures occur in patients older than 65 years old. Both fractures are more common in women than in men by a margin of three to one. Other risk factors include white race, neurological impairment, malnutrition, impaired vision, malignancy, and decreased physical activity. Osteoporosis, although present in the population at risk, has not been shown to be more prevalent in patients with fractures than in age-matched controls. The average age of patients who sustain a femoral neck fracture is 3 years younger than that of those with trochanteric fracture. Most patients with femoral neck fractures have sustained a low-energy injury. Only a few injuries involve major (high-impact) trauma.

In the case of young individuals who sustain a femoral neck fracture, the resultant trauma is major, usually resulting in a direct force along the shaft of the femur, with or without a rotational component. The increased magnitude of trauma leads to more marked soft tissue devascularization and comminution, which give rise to the increased incidence of treatment failure in young adults. The other mechanism of injury in this age-group is a stress fracture seen in runners and military recruits.

	Fracture Neck of femur	**Trochantric Fracture**
Age	Fracture of little younger age than trochantric	Seen In later ages
Trauma	Relatively high velocity trauma	Trivial trauma
Site of fracture	Mostly intracapsular	Always extra capsular
Deformity (shortning & external rotation	Less pronounced	More pronounced

Management	Prosthetic replacement in elderly Osteosynthesis in younger patients	Managed well with osteosynthesis
Complication	Non-union / AVN	Malunion

If the diagnosis of a hip fracture is questionable in an acutely painful hip, bone scanning and MRI have shown excellent sensitivity in identifying these injuries.

Classification of fracture neck of femur

- **Garden classification (1961)** – based on
  - Degree of displacement
  - Relates to risk of vascular disruption

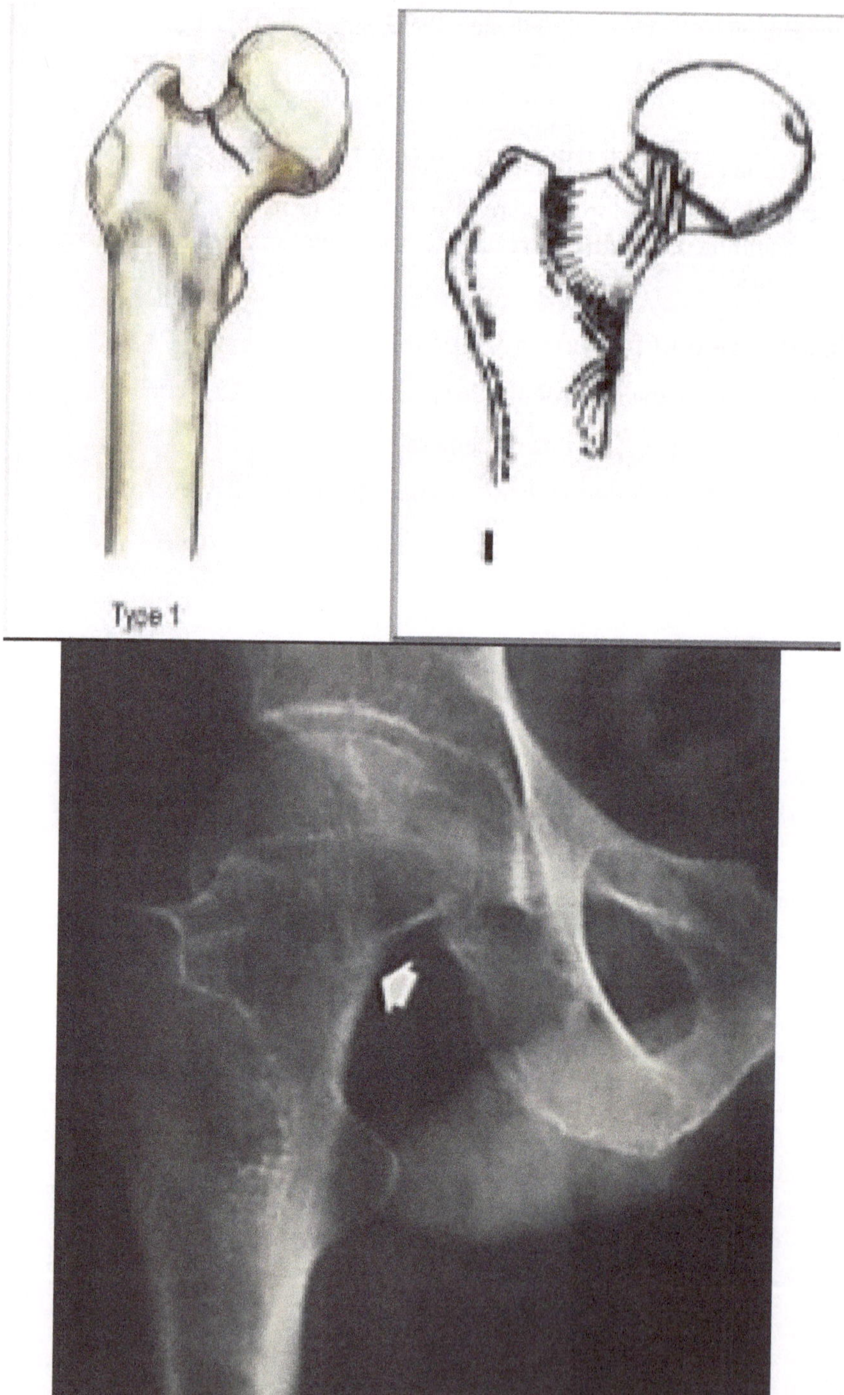

Type 1 - Incomplete fracture (impacted fracture)

Intact inferior neck trabeculae

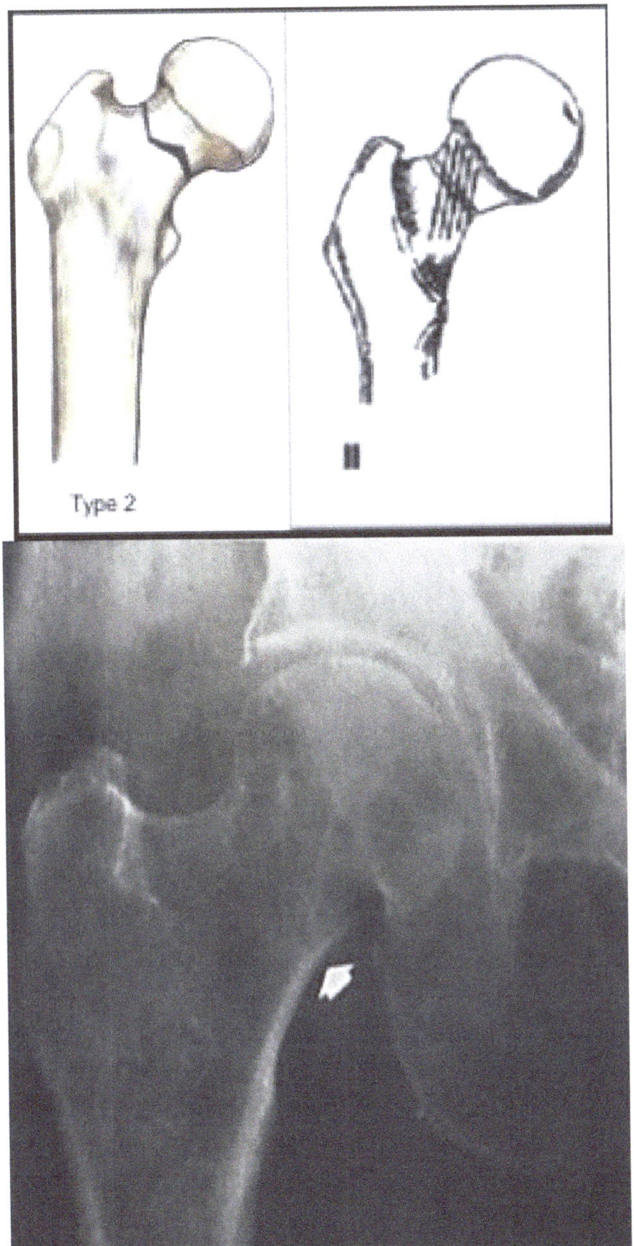

Type 2 : Complete fracture without displacement

Distal fragment trabeculae are in normal alignment

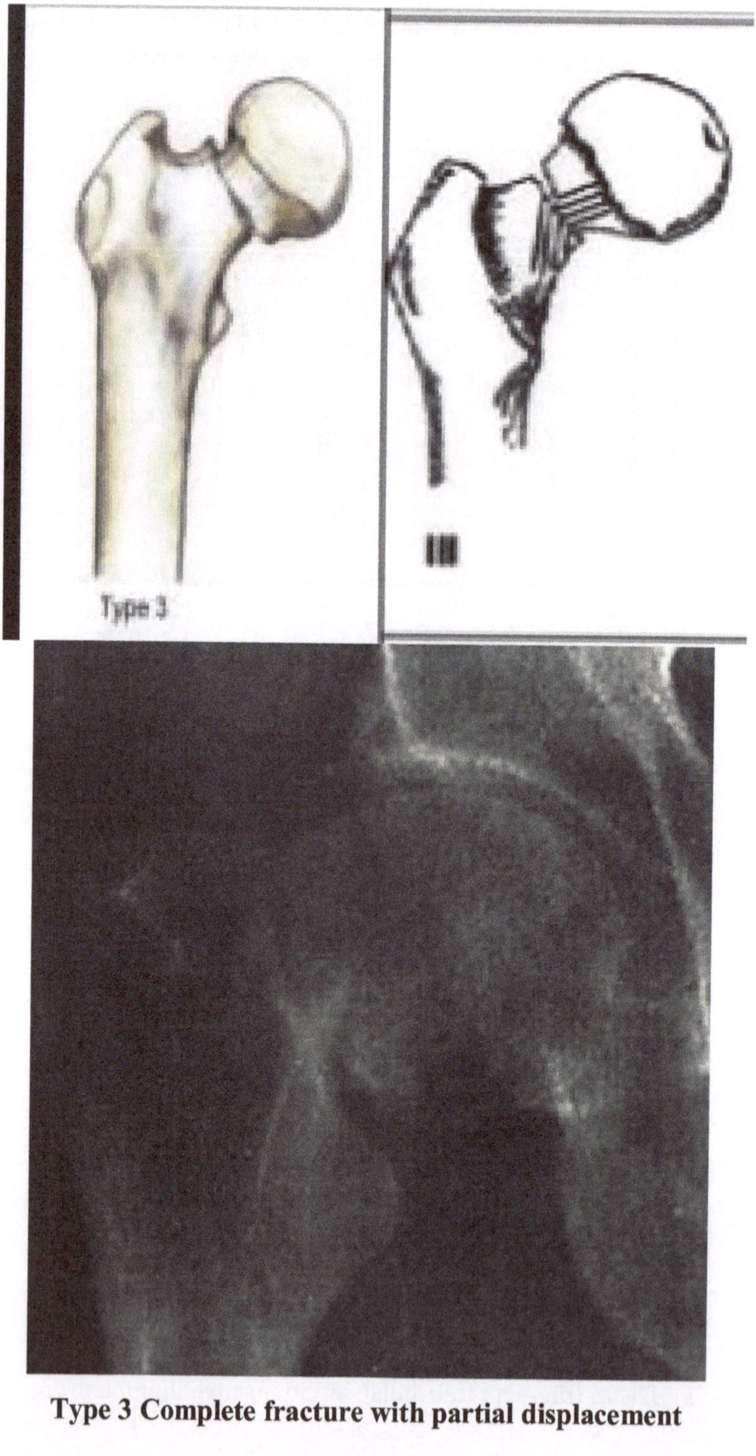

Type 3 Complete fracture with partial displacement

- Intact posterior retinaculum
- Trabecular pattern of femoral head does not line up with that of acetabulum

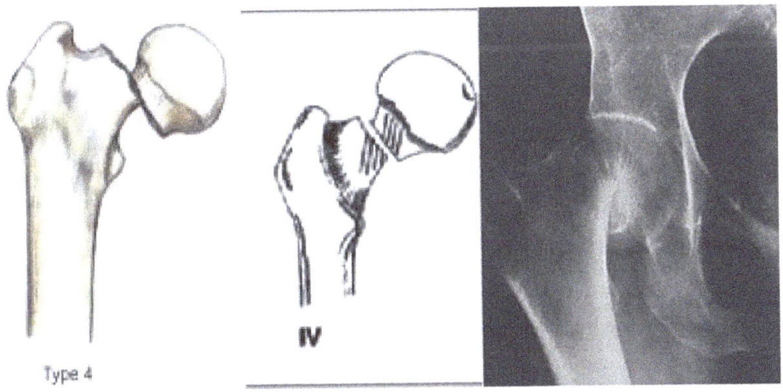

Type 4 Complete fracture with full displacement (trabeculae of the head realign themselves with the trabeculae of the acetabulum)

- Poor interobserver reliability
- Later Modified to:
  - Non-displaced
    - Garden I (valgus impacted)
    - Garden II (non-displaced)
  - Displaced
    - Garden III and IV
- **Pauwels Classification (1935)**
  - Post reduction classification
  - Based on fracture orientation or angle
  - Relates to biomechanical stability
  - More vertical fracture has more shear force hence less stable

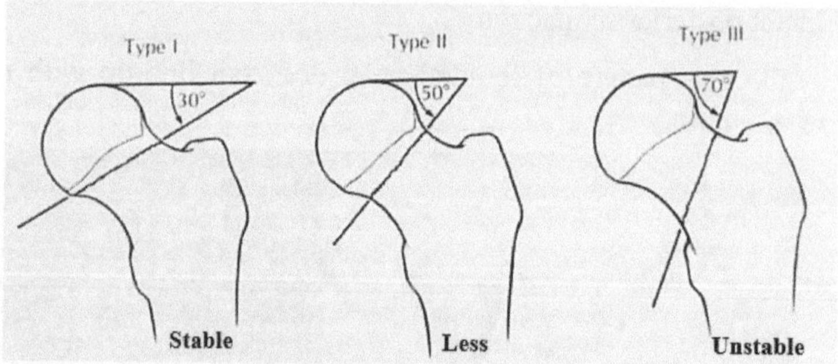

ANATOMICAL CLASSIFICATION

1.Subcapital, 2.Transcervical, 3.Basicervical **Unstable**

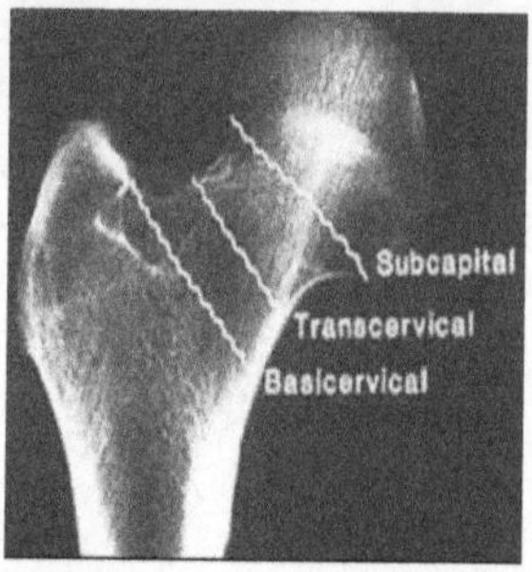

Hip fracture in children

Pediatric hip fractures generally are classified by the method of Delbet because its simplicity and uniformity allow accurate description and reporting of results of each fracture by type.

Type I is a transepiphyseal separation, withoutor withdislocation of the femoral head from the acetabulum.

Type II is a transcervical fracture.

Type III is a cervicotrochanteric fracture.

Type IV is an intertrochanteric fracture

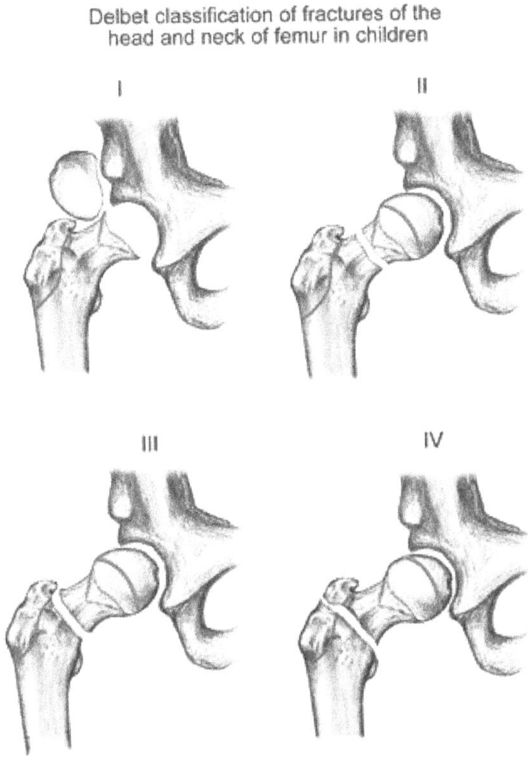

Type I

Fractures in children under 2 or 3 years of age have a better prognosis than in older children. ON is unlikely, although coxa vara, coxa breva, and premature physeal closure can cause subsequent leg length discrepancy

Type II

Transcervical fractures account for 46% of fractures of the head and neck of the femur in children. The risk of ON is thought by most investigators to be directly related to the initial displacement of the fracture, although a few have hypothesized an intraarticular hemarthrosis with tamponade as the etiology of vascular impairment.

Type III

Cervicotrochanteric fractures are, by definition, located at or above the anterior intertrochanteric line and are the second most common type of hip fracture in children, representing about 34% of fractures. The incidence of ON is 20% to 30%, and, as in type II fractures, the risk of ON is directly related to the degree of displacement at the time of injury. Premature physeal closure occurs in 25% of patients and coxavara in 14%. Displaced type III fractures are similar to type II fractures in regard to the development of complications. Nondisplaced type III fractures have a much lower complication rate than displaced fractures.

Type IV

Intertrochanteric fractures account for only 12% of fractures of the head and neck of the femur in children. This fracture has the lowest complication rate of all four types. Nonunion and ON after this fracture are rare. Coxa vara and premature physeal closure have occasionally been reported

Management Fracture Neck Femur

In Paediatric age group

Type I fracture treatment is based on the age of the child and fracture stability after reduction.

In toddlers under 2 years of age with nondisplaced or minimally displaced fractures, simple spica cast immobilization is likely to be successful. Because the fracture tends to displace into varus and external rotation, the limb should be casted in mild abduction and neutral rotation to prevent displacement.

Displaced fractures in toddlers should be reduced closed by gentle traction, abduction, and internal rotation. If the fracture locks on and is stable, casting without fixation is indicated.

If the fracture is not stable, it should be fixed with small smooth pins that access the femoral neck and cross the physis. If casting without fixation is done, repeat x-rays should be taken within days to look for displacement, because the likelihood of successful repeat reduction decreases rapidly with time and healing in a young child.

Children older than 2 years should always have operative fixation even if the fracture is undisplaced because the complications of late displacement may be great. Smooth pins can be used in young children, but cannulated screws are better for older, larger children. Fixation should cross the physis into the capital femoral epiphysis. Irreducibility mandates an open reduction and internal fixation. Postoperative spica cast immobilization is mandatory in all but the oldest and most reliable adolescents. Fixation may be removed shortly after fracture healing to enable further growth in younger patients.

Closed reduction of type IB fracture dislocations may be attempted, but immediate open reduction is necessary if a single attempt at closed reduction is unsuccessful. Internal fixation is mandatory. The surgical approach should be from the side to which the head is dislocated, generally posterolateral. Parents must be advised in advance about the risk of ON.

Type II and Type III

Displaced neck fractures should always be treated with anatomic reduction and stable internal fixation to minimize the risk of late complications. In two large series, the prevalences of coxa vara and nonunion were high in displaced transcervical fractures treated with immobilization but without internal fixation.

Much lower prevalences of these two complications have been documented in patients treated with anatomic closed or open reduction and internal fixation.

Internal fixation also is recommended by most investigators for nondisplaced transcervical fractures because the risk of late displacement in such fractures far outweighs the risk of percutaneous screw fixation, especially in young children.

Nondisplaced type II fractures in children under 5 years of age can be managed with spica casting and close follow-up but fixation remains preferable. Even then, close follow-up is necessary to prevent varus displacement in the cast.

If possible, screws should be inserted short of the physis in type III fractures; however, if physeal penetration is necessary for purchase, it must be done. The risks of premature physeal closure and trochanteric overgrowth are much less than those of nonunion, pin breakage, and ON. Treatment of the fracture is the first priority, and any subsequent growth disturbance and leg length discrepancy are secondary.

Nondisplaced cervicotrochanteric fractures can be treated adequately in an abduction one-and-one-half spica cast with close follow-up .Displaced cervicotrochanteric fractures have been shown to have a complication rate similar to that for type II fractures and should be treated similarly. Fixation generally does not need to cross the physis in type III fractures.

In a more distal cervicotrochanteric fracture, especially in a child over 5 years of age, a pediatric hip compression screw can be used for more secure fixation. Consideration may be given to capsulotomy or aspiration of the joint to eliminate tense hemarthrosis at the time of surgery. Spica casting is routine, except in older reliable children. Hardware removal at 6 to 12 months after fracture union will avoid bony overgrowth of the hardware.

MANAGEMENT IN ADULTS

Management in adults depends upon a lot of factors that incudes.

a. Age of the patient (physiological age is more important)
b. Displacement of fracture
c. Pre fracture ambulatory status
d. Previous hip pathology

There is a broad universal protocol for management of fracture neck of femur in adults considering above mentioned parameters

1. ***Patient with physiological age >65 years***

   a. **Undisplaced imapcted fracture** → Good bone stock and community ambulatory – Trial of insitu fixation with dynamic hip screw can be taken with explained prognosis

   ↓ Poor bone quality or home bound ambulatory-hemiarthroplasty will be management.

   b. **Displaced fracture** → Irrespective of bone quality – previously healthy hip-hemiarthroplasty
   Arthritic hip – Total hip arthroplasty

2. ***Patient younger than 65-***

   a. **Undisplaced fracture** → Insitu fixation CCS

   b. **Displaced fracture** → Closed reduction manoeuvre
   ↓ Reducible → ↓ Fixation with CCS/DHS reduction
   → Irreducible → ↓ Open → ↓ CCS/DHS

Closed reduction techniques

A femoral neck fracture with minimal displacement can usually be reduced in extension on the fracture table

Whitman described a reduction method that involved traction on the limb in extension followed by internal rotation and abduction

The fractured extremity is tied to footplate in an externally rotated position→ with the extremity externally rotated, it is abducted approximately 20* → Traction is applied→the extremity is internally rotated until the patella is internally rotated 20 - 30*.

If this Whitmanmethod fails or if significant displacement remains, a reduction in flexion should be performed. The hip is flexed to 90 degrees and the leg externally rotated. Traction plus external rotation should be applied while the hip is then gently extended and internally rotated. Extension is combined with internal rotation of the femur. This procedure disengages the fracture fragments in flexion, reduces the fracture with extension and reengages the fracture segment in internal rotation.

Leadbetter championed the reduction of femoral neck in full hip flexion. In this technique, the affected leg is flexed at the hip to 90 degrees and traction (with slight adduction of the femoral shaft) is applied along the axis of the femur. In this position, the thigh is rotated internally. The leg then is circumducted into abduction (maintaining internal rotation) and brought down to table level in extension. Leadbetter evaluated the reduction with the so-called heel/palm test, in which the heel is placed in the palm of an outstretched hand. If reduction is complete, the leg will not rotate spontaneously externally.

Reduction assessment

GARDEN'S INDEX **- In X-ray antero posterior view**

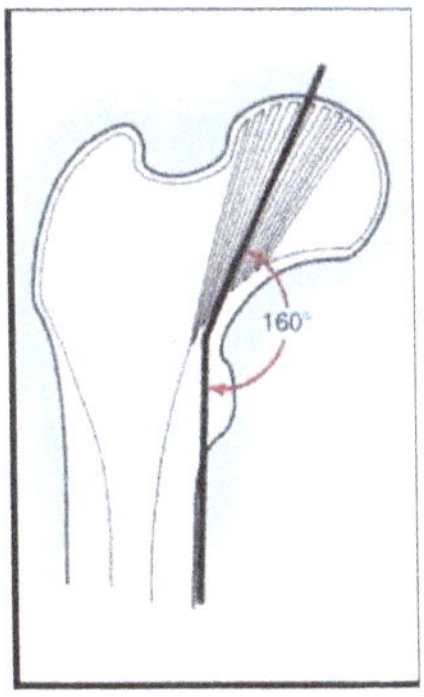

- Angle formed by the central axis of the medial trabecular system in the head fragment and the medial cortex of the femoral shaft should be 160-180*
- Angle < 160* denotes varus reduction
- Angle > 180* denotes valgus reduction

In X-ray lateral view

- Major trabeculae are in the same axis as axis of femoral neck or lie at an angle of 180*

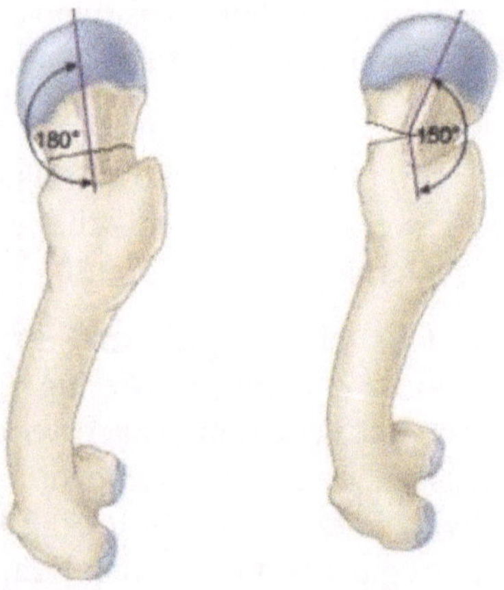

• Alignment index < 155* or > 180* increases incidence of Avascular necrosis

Impacted fractures must be distinguished from nondisplaced fractures of the neck of the femur. Impacted fracture surfaces are crushed together or invaginated so that the trabeculae and usually the cortex of the neck are pushed into the soft trabecular bone of the head. This impaction imparts a significant amount of stability at the fracture site and suggests a conservative or nonoperative approach. Despite this apparent stability, it is far more certain and safer to fix these fractures with multiple screws because almost 100% of impacted fractures unite, but 15% or more displace if not stabilized by multiple screw fixation. In nondisplaced fractures of the femoral neck (Garden stage II), there is no impaction and no stability, and almost all subsequently displace if not internally fixed. Rates of nonunion and osteonecrosis for nondisplaced fractures are low when these fractures are treated with multiple screw fixation.

Nonoperative Treatment

Operative management consisting of fracture reduction and stabilization, which permits early patient mobilization and minimizes many of the complications of prolonged bedrest, has become the treatment of choice for most femoral neck fractures. There nevertheless remain situations in which surgery cannot be performed and treatment must be nonoperative. One example involves the elderly person whose medical condition carries an excessively high risk of mortality from anesthesia and surgery (for example, one who has sustained a recent myocardial infarction). Nonambulatory patients who have minimal discomfort following fracture should also be treated nonoperatively and permitted early bed-to-chair mobilization. If a patient with a femoral neck fracture is to be treated nonoperatively, the patient should be taken out of bed to chair once pain permits with acceptance of any proximal femoral deformity.

Our emphasis in this book has been on hemiarthroplasty using specially bipolar certain points are worth mentioning about hemiarthroplasty in fracture neck of femur.

Relative indications for hemiarthroplasty are as follows:

1.Advanced physiological age. Prosthetic replacement probably should be reserved for patients 65 years old or older with a life expectancy of no more than 10 to 15 years has become a old saying now. With advancement in design of bipolar prosthesis like the one developed at our department at BHU (BHU Bipolar) bipolar hemiarthroplasy now have a broader indication profile and can be used in middle aged patients and moderately arthritic hip as suggested in various studies conducted over a long duration.

2. Fracture-dislocation of the hip in an older patient. If the fracture involves the superior weight bearing surface of the head, the insertion of a prosthesis is preferable to closed treatment or open reduction of the fragment. If a substantial fragment of the inferior part of the head is fractured, the dislocation should be reduced promptly and, if the head fragment is not caught in the joint, treated closed; if necessary, open reduction of the hip can be performed, and the fragment can be removed. Such treatment results in a good hip if the superior weight bearing surface of the head is intact.

Stronger indications for hemiarthroplasty include the following:

1. A fracture that cannot be satisfactorily reduced or fixed with stability, especially with posterior comminution.

2. Femoral neck fractures that lose fixation several weeks after operation.

3. Some pre-existing lesions of the hip. In patients with pre-existing lesions, an arthroplasty already may have been indicated, and the fracture merely makes the decision immediate. Patients with osteonecrosis of the head of the femur from unknown causes, from irradiation, or from a previous dislocation and patients with severe rheumatoid or degenerative arthritis of the hip probably would have a better hip after insertion of prosthesis than before the fracture.

4. Malignancy. A malignancy may be an indication for the insertion of a prosthesis. A patient with a short life expectancy, whether the fracture is pathological or primarily the result of trauma, is best treated with a prosthesis. If the fracture is pathological, the insertion of a prosthesis offers not only a good solution, but also an opportunity to perform an open biopsy and to establish a definite diagnosis. In pathological fractures, supplementing the fixation with methylmethacrylate usually provides sufficient stability.

5. Neurological disorders. Patients subject to uncontrolled epileptic seizures and patients with severe uncontrolled parkinsonism are treated better with a primary prosthesis. Many of these disorders are controllable, however, and the indication may not always be absolute.

6. Old, undiagnosed fractures of the femoral neck. Occasionally, a fracture of the femoral neck goes undiscovered for several weeks. Sometimes multiple injuries may delay treatment of a fractured femoral neck even after its diagnosis. An untreated, unreduced, and unimpacted fracture of the femoral neck that is more than 3 weeks old should have a primary prosthesis, other things being equal.

7. Fracture of the neck of the femur with complete dislocation of the femoral head. This lesion is rare and is best treated by primary prosthetic replacement because osteonecrosis of the head is certain under these circumstances.

8. A patient who probably cannot withstand two operations. If a patient's general condition prohibits a second operation, a primary prosthesis is justified.

9. Patients with psychoses or mental deterioration. Elderly patients with fractures of the femoral neck often already have Alzheimer disease, and protected weight bearing in such patients may be unreliable, with immediate unprotected weight bearing resulting in possible loss of fixation, especially in severely comminuted fractures. A primary prosthesis may be justified in these circumstances.

Non union in fracture neck of femur

Femoral neck fractures usually are entirely intracapsular, and, common to all intracapsular fractures, the synovial fluid bathing the fracture may interfere with the healing process.

Because the femoral neck essentially has no periosteal layer, all healing must be endosteal. Angiogenic-inhibiting factors in synovial fluid also can inhibit fracture repair.

These factors, along with the precarious blood supply to the femoral head, make healing unpredictable and nonunions fairly frequent.

With anatomical reduction and stable fixation, the incidence of nonunion should be acceptably low.

Management in case of elderly patient will be a hemiarthroplasty , while in case of a young patient with prolonged life expectancy valgus osteotomy needs to be performed(depending upon viability of head).

Avascular Necrosis

As with nonunion, the development of osteonecrosis correlates with the extent of initial trauma and the displacement of the fracture, with some question concerning the tamponading effect of the intracapsular hematoma.

Tearing the capsular vessels the injury deprives the head its main blood supply.Intra articular bone has only flimsy periosteum and no contact with soft tissue.

Prompt reduction of the displacement possibly may open some of the retinacular vessels that are temporarily closed by kinking or stretching, and rigid fixation may permit reestablishment of some vascular continuity that otherwise might not be preserved if reduction and fixation are delayed

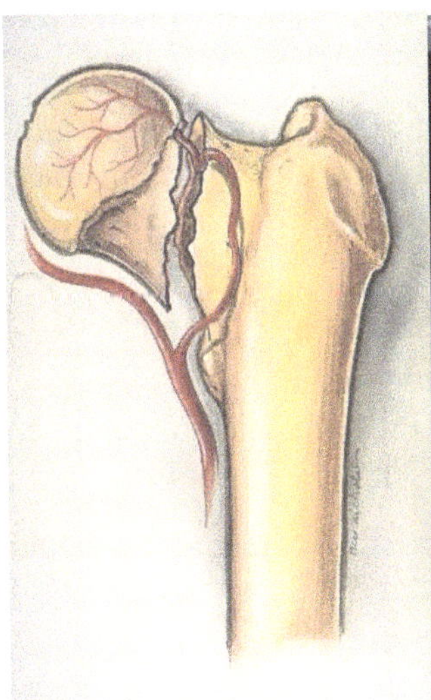

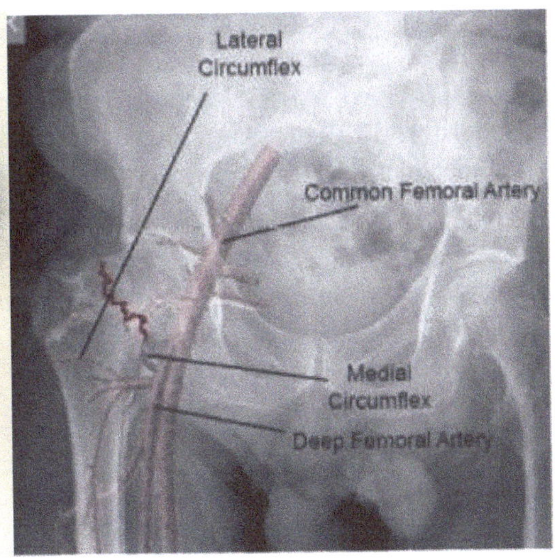

Management is guided by symptoms : In **early cases where x ray changes are not evident** Young patients can be managed with protected weight bearing and core decompression when needed.

Elderly patient might go for prosthesis placement or Girdlestone arthroplsty.

In **latecases with x ray changes** - Prosthesis placement remains the option.

REFERENCES

1. Canale & Beaty: Campbell's Operative Orthopaedics, 11th ed. Mosby, An Imprint of Elsevier2007
2. Chapman, Michael W. Chapman's Orthopaedic Surgery, 3rd Edition, Lippincott Williams & Wilkins2001.
3. Bucholz, Robert W.; Heckman, James D.; Court-Brown, Charles M. Rockwood & Green's Fractures in Adults, 6th Edition, Lippincott Williams & Wilkins2006.
4. Beaty, James H.; Kasser, James R. Rockwood & Wilkins' Fractures in Children, 6th Edition, Lippincott Williams & Wilkins2006.
5. Sevitt S, Thompson RG. Distribution and anastomosis of arteries supplying the head of the femur. J Bone Joint Surg (Br).1966; 47 : 560-573.
6. Dedrick DK, Mackenzie JR, Burney RE. Complications of femoral neck fracture in young adults. J Trauma. 1986 Oct;26(10):932-7.
7. Avery PP, Baker RP, Walton MJ, Rooker JC, Squires B, Gargan MF, Bannister GC. Total hip replacement and hemiarthroplasty in mobile, independent patients with a displaced intracapsular fracture of the femoral neck: a seven- to ten-year follow-up report of a prospective randomised controlled trial. J Bone Joint Surg Br. 2011 Aug;93(8)
8. Kazley JM, Banerjee S, Abousayed MM, Rosenbaum AJ. Classifications in Brief: Garden Classification of Femoral Neck Fractures. Clin. Orthop. Relat. Res. 2018 Feb;476(2):441-445
9. Koval KJ, Zuckerman JD. Hip Fractures: I. Overview and Evaluation and Treatment of Femoral-Neck Fractures. J Am Acad Orthop Surg. 1994 May;2(3):141-149.
10. Protzman RR, Burkhalter WE. Femoral-neck fractures in young adults. J Bone Joint Surg Am. 1976 Jul;58(5):689-95.

HISTORY OF HIP ARTHROPLSTY

Over the last three centuries, treatment of hip arthritides has evolved from rudimentary surgery to modern total hip arthroplasty (THA), which is considered one of the most successful surgical interventions ever developed. An evaluation of such past enterprises is relevant, and reminds us how medical research and procedures are not isolated developments, but correlate to the social, economical, and cultural framework of their time.

EARLY HIP ARTHRITIS SURGERY IN THE 1800s

Toward the end of the eighteenth century, the field of operative orthopaedics was considerably advanced as a result of the progress made in identifying the physiology of the skeletal tissues. Excision of the joints was practiced liberally for many types of joint diseases. **Henry Park (1744-1831)** worked at The Royal Infirmary of Liverpool United Kingdom made a special name in the beginning.

As with all surgical innovations enthusiasm shown at that time for joint excision was the result of special circumstances, and off course it was in reaction to the appalling frequency with which amputation was being practiced in Europe and America. Liverpool was a large commercial port and sailors used to arrive with wounded limbs and in many instances injured months before. These types of injuries required a radical treatment, which in the late 1700s meant amputation.

Amputation of the extremity in these cases often offered a simple but, unnecessary solution to the problem, as Park thought. However, the technical ease of amputation when compared to joint excision slowed the acceptance of this technique by Park's colleagues. During the pre-anesthesia era, rapidity of a procedure was most valued.

Anthony White[i] **(1782-1849)** of the Westminster Hospital in London, carried out the first excision arthroplasty in 1821 though he did not make a personal report of the operation. This procedure ameliorated pain and preserved mobility, but at the expense of stability.

However, **John Rhea Barton (1794-1871)** in Philadelphia, is credited with performing the first osteotomy on an ankylosed hip **in 1826.** He performed an intertrochanteric osteotomy without anesthesia in only seven minutes. After twenty days, he manipulated the extremity to provoke a fibrous reaction at the ends of the severed bone, and thus created a pseudarthrosis. Three months after the operation, the patient walked reasonably well with a cane, but six years later all motion had been lost. Barton provided the first evidence that motion would prevent the fusion of bone. This popularized hip osteotomy as a rational plan for overcoming bony ankylosis, an untreated lesion till that time. However, although there were some spectacular successes, the outcome was generally discomfortingly unpredictable. Most of the operated joints eventually became ankylosed, a disappointing outcome for such a perilous procedure that had a mortality rate of approximately 50 percent, high even by the day's standards.

Auguste Stanislas Verneuil (1823–95), from Paris, France, performed soft tissue hip interpositions in **1860.** Work of **Léopold Ollier's** (1830-1900) at the Hôtel-Dieu hospital in Lyon, France, generated tremendous interest in the concept of interpositional arthroplasty. In **1885**, he described the interposition of adipose tissue in uninfected joints. However, he did not fix the interposed material to the subjacent bone and his procedures were generally ineffective. Czech surgeon **Vitezlav Chlumsky** (1867-1943), working in Breslau, Germany systematically experimented with many interpositional materials. Among the wide variety of materials he used was muscle, celluloid, silver plates, rubber struts, magnesium, zinc, glass, pyres, decalcified bones, wax and celluloid.

Berliner Professor **Themistocles Glück** (1853-1942) led the way in the development of hip implant fixation. In **1891,** Glück produced an ivory, ball and socket joint that he fixed to bone with nickel-plated screws. Subsequently, he experimented with a mixture of plaster of Paris, and powdered pumice with resin to provide fixation. Glück was also a pioneer in proposing the idea of biocompatibility, which explains how a foreign material placed in the body must be well tolerated by the patient's body.

INTERPOSITIONAL HIP ARTHROPLASTY IN THE 1900s

Earlier in the 1900s, Murphy, along with **Erich Lexer** (1867-1937) from München, Germany, had advocated the hip interposition of *fascia lata.* Other interesting interpositional material was introduced at the turn of nineteenth century by a French surgeon, **Foedre** (b. ca. 1860), who noted that pig bladder was sufficiently strong to withstand the stresses of weight bearing and intra-articular pressure. By **1918, William Steven Baer** (1872-1931) had popularized pig bladder arthroplasty at the Johns Hopkins Hospital.

In **1925,** a surgeon in Boston, Massachusetts, **M.N. Smith-Petersen**, M.D., molded a piece of glass into the shape of a hollow hemisphere which could fit over the ball of the hip joint and provide a new smooth surface for movement. Smith-Petersen had observed a smooth membrane around an excised piece of glass during an unrelated procedure. Encouraged by this finding he designed this mould. He also described the anterior surgical approach to the hip for use in this procedure, which bears his name. While proving biocompatibility, the glass could not withstand the stress of walking and quickly failed.

EARLY PROSTHETIC HIP ARTHROPLASTY IN THE 1900

The first to use a rubber femoral prosthesis was at **Pierre Delbet** (1861-1925) at La Ferté Gaucher, Departement Seine-et-Marne, France. He used a rubber femoral prosthesis in **1919** to replace one-half of the hip joint.

However, a lot of attention for early prostheses was garnered by the **Judet brothers - Robert (1901-80) and Jean (1905-95)**, from Paris, France. They used an acrylic prosthesis **in 1948**. The Judet prostheses turned out to be exceptionally susceptible to wear, and failed even before the general acclaim had ceased.

In the 1940s, resection of the femoral head, especially for tuberculosis and infection, was popularized by Gathorne Robert Girdlestone (1881-1950) from the military orthopaedic center, The radical excision arthroplasty that bears his name is occasionally used today as last resort in failed THA, a procedure that is called "conversion to a Girldestone".

The Judet brothers' concept was refined by **Frederick Röeck Thompson**, (1907-83) and Austin Moore (1899-1963) who developed a Vitallium prosthesis Dr. Moore inserted the first such metal prosthesis at John Hopkins Hospital in 1940. The procedure replaced the proximal twelve inches of a femur, destroyed by a recurrent giant cell tumor, with a custom made Vitallium prosthesis.

In 1938, **Philip Wiles (1899-1966)** of the Middelsex Hospital in London described the first THA using precisely fitted stainless steel components which were fixed to the bone with screws and bolts. However, he did not achieve satisfactory results.

Peter Ring (b. 1922), working in parallel with the Russians, in Redhill, Surrey, started his clinical experience with cementless components with a metal-on-metal articulation in 1964. Some of his early arthroplasties provided surprisingly good results with up to 97% of implants surviving at 17 years of follow up. Both the McKee-Farrar and the Ring models were abandoned in the 1970s in favour of Charnley's model, which turned out to be the most successful model as far as THA is concerned till date.

An awareness of the history of hip arthroplasty is necessary to appreciate not only its current status but also its future.

Timeline on Hip Arthroplasty

1827 - John Rhea Barton moved a subtrachanteric osteotomy early to create a false joint.

1867 - Louis Ollier studied joint repair after damage.

1885 - Ollier's book on joint resection raises much interest in interpositional arthroplasty, and many tissues and material are tried without much success.

1894 - Themistocles Gluck : Ivory replacement of upper tibia and hip replacement with an ivory ball.

1894 - Jules Pean : Prosthelic replacement of tuberculous shoulder. Pean went on to design hip and knee replacements.

1902 - John Murphy uses fat and fascia as interposition for arthroplasty.

1903 - Delbert – Hip replacement

1917 - William Baer reports on 100 patients using allograft interposition in Baltimore.

1921 - Putti uses all kinds of interposition in Italy

1923 - Hey Groves replaces hip with ivory ball and stem

1923 - Marius Smith – Petersen starts developing a mold arthroplasty, first using glass and later vitallium

1937 - Methyl Methacrylate marketed as Plexiglass

1938 - Philip Wiles replaces both the femoral head and acetabulum with a metal prosthesis in six patients

1940 - McKee makes models of a hip prosthesis but war stops him from trying it out. In 1951 he reports 3 patients. He continues to improve the design of his metal-on-metal prosthesis until he retires and the advantages of metal on plastic become clearer.

1943 - Austin Moore and Harold Bohlman : Femoral head replacement for tumour. The original design has side plates but later they introduce the idea of an intramedullary stem.

1946 - Robert and Jean Judet develop mushroom shaped femoral head prosthesis. The material is acrylic, which breaks; and the stem - following the axis of the neck - is biomechanically unsound.

1950 - Charnley starts to develop hip replacement but gives up in favour of arthrodesis.

1951 - McKee and Farrar describe a metal-on-metal replacement in Norwich.

1952 - FR Thompson : Femoral head replacement.

1953 - Edouard Harboush in New-York uses dental cement to hold a hip prosthesis and a cup in place.

1954 - John Charnley hears a squeaking Judet's prosthesis and hits on the idea of low friction arthroplasty.

1961 - Charnley's report in the Lancet.

1962 - High density polyethylene.

1964 - Peter Ring : Metal-on-metal cementless replacement with a screw in the acetabulum

1968 - The Hip Society established under the leadership of Frank Stinchfield.

1970 - Ceramic surfaces introduced by Hulbert.

1973 - Porous coating – Food and drug administration approves the use of acrylic cement.

1974 - Bateman introduced the concept of the bipolar or universal endoprosthesis. An intermediate step between the Moore type of endoprosthesis and a total hip system.

1985 - Giliberty reported the bipolar.

REFERENCES

1. MacLennan WJ. History of arthritis and bone rarefaction: evidence from paleopathology onwards. Scot Med J. 1999;44:18–20

2. Rogers J, Watt I, Dieppe P. Arthritis in Saxon and mediaeval skeletons. Br Med J. (Clin Res Ed) 1981;283(6307):1668–1670.

3. Thould AK, Thould BT. Arthritis in Roman Britain. Br Med J. (Clin Res Ed) 1983 Dec 24;287(6409):1909–1911.

4. Trinkaus E. Pathology and the posture of the La Chapelle-aux-Saints Neandertal. Am J Phys Anthropol. 1985 Jun;67(1):19–41.

5. Park H. An account of a new method of treating diseases of the joints of the knee and elbow. In: Pott MP, editor. London: 1782.
6. Bilguer JH. De membrorum amputatione rarissime admnistranda. 1761.
7. Leonardo RA. History of Surgery. New York: Froben Press; 1943. 237 p
8. Anthony White (Obituary) Lancet. 1849;1:324.
9. Barton JR. On the treatment of anchylosis, by the formation of artificial joints. North Amer Med and Surg Jour. 1827 Jan–Feb;3(279):400.
10. Stanley P. For Fear of Pain, British Surgery, 1790-1850. Amsterdam: Editions Rodopi BV; 2003.
11. Ollier L. Traité des Résections et des opérations conservatives qu'ont peut practiquere surle sistême osseux. Paris: 1885.
12. Chlumsky V. Zentralblatt für or thopaedische Chirurgie. 1896. Continued Centralblatt für orthopaedische Chirurgie un mechanik from 1887-1890.
13. Rang M. Anthology of Orthopaedics. Edinburgh, London, New York: Churchill Livingstone; 1966
14. Murphy JB. Surgical Clinics of Jhon B Murphy. IV. Philadelphia: Sanders; 1915. Cheilotomy
15. Murphy JB. Trans Amer Surg Ass. 1904;22:213.
16. Lexer E. Über Gelenktrasportation. Med Klin Berlin. 1908;4:817.
17. Helferich H. Über Muskeltransplantation beim Menschen. 1882. Paper presented at: Verhandlungen der deutschen Gesellschaft für orthopaedische Chirurgie.
18. Helferich H. Über Operationene an der Kniescheibe. Arch f klin Chir. 1894;48:864.
19. Foedre Zentralbl f Chir. 1896. p. 5.
20. Baer WS. Preliminary report of animal membrane in producing mobility in ankylosed joints. Amer Jour Orth Surg. 1909.
21. Baer WS. Arthroplasty with the aid of animal membrane. Amer Jour Orth Surg. 1918;16(1):171.
22. Jones R, Lovett RW. Orthopaedic. Baltimore: Wm Wood; 1929
23. Whitman R. The Reconstruction Operation for Arthritis Deformans of the Hip. Joint Ann Surg. 1924;80:779.

24. Smith-Petersen M. Evolution of mould arthroplasty of the hip joint. J Bone Joint Surg. (Br) 1948;30(B1):59.
25. Judet J, Judet R. The use of an artificial femoral head for arthroplasty of the hip joint. J Bone Joint Surg. (Br) 1950;32B:166–173
26. Darwin Francis. Oxford University Press; [Accessed 02-05, 2004].
27. Girdlestone GR. The classic. Acute pyogenic arthritis of the hip: an operation giving free access and effective drainage. GR Girdlestone, 1943. Clin Orthop. 1982. Nov, pp. 3–7.
28. Seddon HJ. Oxford University Press; [Accessed 1 Jul, 2004]. Girdlestone, Gathorne Robert (1881-1950) Available at:
29. Bhandari M, Busse JW, Jackowski D, et al. Association between industry funding and statistically significant pro-industry findings in medical and surgical randomized trials. Cmaj. 2004 Mar 17;170(4):477–480.
30. Thompson FR. Vitallium intramedullary hip prosthesis- preliminary report. NY State J Med. 1952;52:3011–3020.
31. Moore AT, Böhlman HR. The classic.Metal hip joint.A case report.By Austin T Moore and Harold R Bohlman. 1943. Clin Orthop. 1983. Jul, pp. 3–6.
32. Wiles P. The Surgery of the osteo-arthritic hip. Br J surg. 1957;45:488–497
33. McKee GK, Watson-Farrar J. Replacement of arthritic hips by the McKee-Farrar prosthesis. J Bone Joint Surg. (Br) 1966;48(2):245–259.
34. Ring PA. Replacement of the hip joint. Ann R Coll Surg Engl. 1971 Jul;48(6):344–355.
35. Gomez PF; Morcuende JA (2005). "Early attempts at hip arthroplasty—1700s to 1950s". Iowa Orthop J.

BIPOLAR ANAESTHESIA

Approximately 98% of hip fractures are managed surgically, as surgery provides better chance of rehabilitation, and reduces the risk of complications. Management of orthopedic patient is different from general surgical patients in many aspects considering age, co-morbidities and the medicines being taken by patient. There is a triad of challenges, faced differently by the patient, the surgeon and the anesthesiologist. The patient is mostly worried about pain, mobility and complications. The surgeon concerned about of intraoperative bleeding, muscles relaxation and the postoperative outcome in terms of bone union or deformity correction. The anesthesiologist faces the challenges throughout the perioperative period. A careful preoperative examination, optimization of any co-morbid condition, safe intraoperative anesthetic techniques, with plan of postoperative pain relief results best outcome. Postoperative physiotherapy results early recovery, early mobilization, and low morbidity and mortality.

Preoperative assessment is essential to check other injuries, coexisting deformities and pre-existing medical problems such as diabetes, hypertension, heart disease, renal, or endocrine disease as decreased organ function and minimal reserve, might challenge the competence of the anesthesiologist. A proper history of drugs intake (antiplatelet agents, anticoagulants and NSAID's), past history of surgery (CABG, stents or permanent pacemakers etc.) is necessary as it poses additional problems. Due to severe pain and trauma cardio respiratory reserve assessment can be difficult in some patients. Previously undiagnosed anemia is common as most of the patients are elderly and malnourished thus increased likelihood of blood transfusion, perioperative morbidity and mortality. As per World Health Organization recommendations, Anemia is defined by the level of hemoglobin less than 13g/dl in males and 12g/dl in non-pregnancy females. Anemia prevalence rates rose rapidly to a rate greater than 20% after age of 85 years. The most common causes of anemia in old age patients are nutritional deficiencies (iron, folate, Vitamin B12), chronic renal failure and chronic inflammatory diseases. Early detection, evaluation and preoperative management of anemia are required. As per NATA (Network for Advancement of Transfusion Alternative) recommendations for preoperative major orthopedic surgery.

Recommendation 1: It is recommended that elective surgical patients have a hemoglobin level determination as close to 28 days before the scheduled surgical procedure as possible.

Recommendation 2: It is suggested that the patient's target hemoglobin before elective surgery be within the normal range (> 13g/dl for male, > 12 g/dl for female).

Recommendation 3: It is recommended that laboratory testing be performed to further evaluate anemia for nutritional deficiencies, chronic renal insufficiency, and/or chronic inflammatory disease.

Recommendation 4: It is recommended that nutritional deficiencies be treated.

Recommendation 5: It is suggested that stimulation of erythropoiesis be used for anemic patients in whom nutritional deficiencies have been ruled out, corrected or both (Figure 1)

Transfusion trigger for red cell transfusion in intraoperative period is considered 7g/dl; in postoperative period 8 g/dl and 10 g/dl in patients with coronary artery diseases.

Venous thromboembolism is an important and significant source of morbidity and mortality in orthopedic patients. Nearly all hospitalized patients have at least 1 risk factor for thromboembolism; approximately 40% have 3 or more risk factors (Table 1). The agent, dose and duration of thromboprophylaxis depend on the identification of these risk factors. The perioperative management for the patients on warfarin or antiplatlet therapy has been given in table number 2 and 3.

Table 1: Risk Factors for Venous Thromboembolism

Surgery
Trauma (major trauma or lower-extremity injury)
Immobility, lower-extremity paresis
Cancer (active or occult)
Cancer therapy (hormonal, chemotherapy, angiogenesis inhibitors, radiotherapy)
Venous compression (tumor, hematoma, arterial abnormality)
Previous VTE
Increasing age
Pregnancy and the postpartum period
Estrogen-containing oral contraceptives or hormone replacement therapy
Selective estrogen receptor modulators
Erythropoiesis-stimulating agents
Acute medical illness
Inflammatory bowel disease
Nephrotic syndrome
Myeloproliferative disorders
Paroxysmal nocturnal hemoglobinuria
Obesity
Central venous catheterization
Inherited or acquired thrombophilia

The goal of preoperative assessment is optimization of anemia, elevated blood sugar, blood pressure, electrolytes and INR to normal range and to take informed written consent of high risk (if applicable).

The choice of anesthetic technique depends on patient preference, type of surgery and ASA class of the patient. The decision of regional against general anesthesia has to be made based on risk / benefit ratio. As compared to general anesthesia regional anesthesia has less infection rates, length of hospital stay, postoperative cardiovascular and pulmonary complications. Neuraxial anesthesia provides splendid intraoperative anesthesia, less bleeding, superior postoperative analgesia and facilitates early physical rehabilitation. It also reduces intraoperative and postoperative use of NSAIDs and other opioids. Thus results in less morbidity, mortality and shorter hospital stay. Neuraxial anesthesia reduces stress response to surgery thus decreases the incidence of postoperative hypoxia, PONV and deep venous thrombosis (DVT).

In evaluating pain during the postoperative days after different surgical techniques, prosthetic replacement surgery appears to be one of the most painful surgeries. Visual analogue (pain) scale (VAS) greater than 5-6 during the first postoperative day have been reported. Hence the adequate postoperative analgesia following surgery is necessary.

Table 2 : Perioperative Management of the patients on Warfarin

Preoperative

- Discontinue warfarin at least 5 days before elective procedure
- Assess INR 1–2 d prior to surgery, if >1.5, consider 1–2 mg oral vitamin K
- Reversal for urgent surgery/procedure, consider 2.5–5 mg oral or IV vitamin K; for immediate reversal, consider PCCs, fresh frozen plasma
- Patients at high risk of thromboembolism
  - Bridge with therapeutic SC LMWH (preferred) or IV UFH
  - Last dose of preoperative LMWH administered 24 h before surgery, administer half of the daily dose
  - Intravenous heparin discontinued 4–6 h before surgery
- No bridging necessary for patients at low risk of thromboembolism

Postoperative

- Patients at low risk of thromboembolism
  - Resume warfarin on POD
- Patients at high risk of thromboembolism (who received preoperative bridging therapy)
  - Minor surgical procedure—resume therapeutic LMWH 24 h postoperatively
  - Major surgical procedure—resume therapeutic LMWH 48–72 h postoperatively or administer low-dose LMWH
- Assess bleeding risk and adequacy of hemostasis when considering timing of the resumption of LMWH or UFH therapy

The concept of multimodal analgesia described by Kehlet in 1993, based on the principle of optimize the balance between efficiency and side effects different drugs. Sensitization is central hyperalgesic component that contributes to increase pain intensity, especially under dynamic conditions plays an important role in postoperative pain management. It meant to sustain independently of peripheral nociceptive stimuli and generates post-surgical chronic pain. This central component can be treated or prevented with multimodal analgesics having additive and synergistic effect.

A - Systemic analgesia

Non-opioid analgesia: The combination of several non-opioid drugs allows reduced need for opioids and consecutively their secondary and side effects. Acetaminophen, non-steroidal anti-inflammatory drugs, ketamine and gabapentin can be used. Gabapentin reduces opioid consumption as well asthe postoperative pain at rest and in dynamic conditions. Thus improves functional recovery after orthopedic surgery. It also prevents pruritus induced by intrathecal morphine. Currently international recommendations concerning postoperative analgesia propose to use gabapentin premedication without exceeding one daily dose of 800mg to avoid side effects like sedation or dizziness.

Opioid analgesia

The use of opioids in prosthetic joint replacement surgery is strongly (level III of WHO) recommended. However in elderly patient use of opioids are limited to avoid central and peripherical side effects.

B - Intrathecal and epidural analgesia

Epidural analgesia provides better analgesia at rest as well as during mobilization than analgesia with drugs alone. However, it is not without risk as central blocks created epidural analgesia can induce arterial hypotension, acute retention of urine, infectious complications and headaches. It also has a small benefit in terms of morbidity and mortality and a low profitability on convalescence.

Spinal anesthesia might be used with some adjuvant, such as clonidine, or liposoluble opioids that can potentiate the action of local anesthetics. But longer duration of postoperative analgesia (>12 to 14h) and the use of high doses of drugs exposes too many side effects (sedation, pruritus, nausea and vomiting, acute urinary retention, hypotension).

C - Peripheral analgesia

Blocks and perineural catheters devices:

Perineural blocks are known to minimize the sympathetic response to surgery, reduces postoperative pain especially during mobilization thus improve patient's satisfaction. Femoral nerve block is with single injection is recommended for postoperative analgesia in hip arthroplasty.

Infiltration of local anesthetic

Local infiltration of anesthetic drug can alleviate postoperative pain but the duration and effectiveness of analgesia by infiltration remain insufficient. However volumes and doses of local anesthetic are more important as with loco regional anesthesia exposing to a potential systemic toxicity.

Table 3: Perioperative Management of the patients on Antiplatelet drugs

Patients with coronary stents

- Elective surgery postponed for the following durations if aspirin and thienopyridine (eg, clopidogrel or prasugrel) therapy must be discontinued
    - Bare metal stents: 6 wk
    - Drug-eluting stents: 6 mo
- If surgery cannot be postponed, continue dual antiplatelet therapy throughout perioperative period

Patients at high risk of cardiac events (exclusive of coronary stents)

- Continue aspirin throughout the perioperative period
- Discontinue clopidogrel/prasugrel 5 d prior to surgery
- Resume thienopyridine 24 h postoperatively

Patients at low risk of cardiac events

- Discontinue dual antiplatelet therapy 7–10 d prior to surgery
- Resume antiplatelet therapy 24 h postoperatively

Complications

Most of the surgeons are reluctant to use neuraxial anesthesia due to fear of urinary retention and bladder catheterization in postoperative period. Contrary to prior belief many recent studies shows that patients undergoing hip arthroplasty have a lower risk of urinary retention after neuraxial anesthesia.

The risk of neurological deficit following epidural/spinal hematoma is also frequently quoted as a concern, although this event is rare. Most of these patients were on antiplatelet medications.

Furthermore, it has been shown that peripheral nerve blocks are safe to use even in patients requiring thromboprophylaxis after joint arthroplasty. There has not been any reported perineural hematoma in continuous lumbar plexus, femoral and continuous or single sciatic blocks in approximately 7000 procedures among patients receiving warfarin, aspirin, fondaparinux, dalteparin and enoxaparin. The reported risk has been below 0.04% for general neurological complication of a central nerve blockade and the rate of neuropathy after peripheral nerve block below 3%, with even less leading to permanent nerve damage. There is only one such case report in a review of 16 studies after peripheral nerve block with sample sizes ranging from 20 to 10309 blocks [Table 4].

Table 4: Risk factors and estimated incidence of Spinal Hematoma and Neuraxial Anaesthesia

	Relative Risk of Spinal Hematoma	Estimated Incidence for Epidural Anesthesia	Estimated Incidence for Spinal Anesthesia
No heparin			
Atraumatic	1.00	1:220,000	1:320,000
Traumatic	11.2	1:20,000	1:29,000
With aspirin	2.54	1:150,000	1:220,000
Heparin anticoagulation following neuraxial procedure			
Atraumatic	3.16	1:70,000	1:100,000
Traumatic	112	1:2000	1:2900
Heparin >1 h after puncture	2.18	1:100,000	1:150,000
Heparin <1 h after puncture	25.2	1:8700	1:13,000
With aspirin	26	1:8500	1:12,000

A number of specific regional anesthetic procedures such as psoas compartment block has all advantages as potent analgesia in postoperative period, but also has possibility of severe complications, with risk of intrathecal or intravasal application of cardiotoxic doses of local anesthetics. However use of ultrasound guided block can be safer and further reduces the chances of complication.

The PROSPECT (procedure specific postoperative pain management) workgroup has recommended the use of peripheral nerve blocks as the primary choice for postoperative pain management in patients undergoing total hip arthroplasty, followed by spinal or epidural anesthesia depending on risk factors and co morbidities.

The spinal anesthesia has been found to have significantly reduced early mortality, fewer incidents of deep vein thrombosis, less acute postoperative confusion, a tendency to fewer myocardial infarctions, fewer cases of pneumonia, fatal pulmonary embolism and postoperative hypoxia, as shown in a meta analyses. The general anesthesia and respiratory diseases were identified as significant predictor of morbidity in the study.

Some recent studies suggest that higher perioperative mortality include advanced age, male gender, poor metabolic equivalents, higher ASA grading, poor mental state, multiple comorbidities, dementia or cognitive impairment, diabetes, cancer and cardiac disease.

The type of anesthesia has significant impact on intraoperative blood loss. This effect has primarily been attributed to hemodynamic differences, with lower and more stable blood pressures achieved through regional anesthesia resulting in less blood loss than general anesthesia. Use of nitrous oxide in the anesthetic gas mix during general anesthesia hinder erythropoiesis during endogenous recovery of red blood cells act as a contributing factor.

As type of anesthesia generally affects body temperature, though neuraxial anesthesia seems to impair thermoregulatory control less than general anesthesia and has less chances of perioperative bleeding.

A number of pre-existing risk factors including a history of prior venous thromboembolic event, obesity, delayed ambulation, hyperlipidemia and female sex have been associated with the development of thromboembolism in postoperative period.

Excluding pulmonary complications, the most common causes of perioperative mortality following orthopedic surgery remains cardiovascular events. The regional anesthesia has also been preferred in hip fracture patients with COPD and has been found to be associated with less pulmonary complications in all hip fracture patients.

Bone cement implantation syndrome is one of the major causes of morbidity and mortality in patients undergoing for cemented arthroplasty. Bone cement implantation syndrome is poorly understood phenomenon and having no clear definition it can occur at the time of cementation, prosthesis insertion, and reduction of the joint or, occasionally, limb tourniquet deflation in a patient undergoing cemented bone surgery. Bone cement comprises of two substances glued together. The first substance is a white powder (pearls) in bone cement consists of small particles of pre-polymerized PMMA. The second one is a liquid monomer of methyl methacrylate (MMA). Both substances are mixed together in theatre after the addition of a catalyst that initiates the polymerization of the monomer fluid. When the bone cement hardens, the individual pearls are entrapped and glued within the net of the polymerized monomer, but no chemical binding occurs between the pearls and the polymerized monomer. BCIS is characterized by a number of clinical features including hypoxia, hypotension, loss of consciousness, cardiac arrhythmias, increased pulmonary vascular resistance (PVR), and cardiac arrest.

A classification system for BCIS has been proposed according to its severity as follows:

Grade 1: Moderate hypoxia ($SpO_2 < 94\%$) or a decrease in systolic arterial pressure (SAP>20%).

Grade 2: severe hypoxia ($SpO_2 < 88\%$) or hypotension (decrease in SAP >40%) or unexpected loss of consciousness.

Grade 3: cardiovascular collapse requiring cardiopulmonary resuscitation.

Raised intramedullary pressure is the main causative factor for release of deposits like marrow, fat, cement particles,air, bone particles, and aggregates of platelets and fibrin. It embolizes to the right atrium, right ventricle, and pulmonary artery leads to right heart failure. Prevention of BCISinvolves the identification, assessment and optimization of high-risk patients and their cardiovascular reserve before surgery and appropriate selection of type of prosthesis, surgical procedure, and techniques in order to minimize the risk of cardiovascular complications.

Raised pulmonary artery pressure can normalize in 24 hours so aggressive resuscitation and supportive treatment is essential to reduce the morbidity and mortality. The concentration of inspired oxygen should be 100% when BCIS is suspected. The hypotension should be managed by adequate i.v. fluid therapy, the use of pulmonary vasodilators for reducing PAP, and the use of inotropes (dobutamine and milrinone) to maintain right ventricular contractility. Intraoperative cardiac output monitoring should be done either in the form of non-invasive CO monitoring, such as transoesophageal Doppler imaging and PiCCO (arterial pulse contour analysis), or invasive CO monitoring with the use of a pulmonary artery flotation catheter to guide vascular filling and the use of vasopressors and inotropes. Patients should be managed by intensive care unit team postoperative period.

REFERENCES

1. Taylor JM, Gropper MA. Critical care challenges in orthopedic surgery patients. Crit Care Med. 2006 Sep;34(9):191-19
2. Goodnough LT, Maniatis A, Earnshaw P, Benoni G, Beris P, Bisbe E, Fergusson DA. Detection, evaluation, and management of preoperative anaemia in the elective orthopedic surgical patient: NATA guidelines. Br J Anaesth. 2011; 106: 13-22.
3. Geerts WH, Bergqvist D, Pineo GF, et al. Prevention of venous thromboembolism: American College of Chest Physiciansevidence-based clinical practice guidelines (8th edition). Chest. 2008;133:381S–453S.
4. Gogarten W, Vandermeulen E, van Aken H, Kozek S, Llau JV, Samama CM. Regional anesthesia and antithrombotic agents: recommendations of the European Society of Anesthesiology. Eur J Anaesthesiol. 2010;27:999–1015.
5. Douketis JD, Spyropoulos AC, Spencer FA, et al. Perioperative management of antithrombotic therapy: antithrombotic therapy and prevention of thrombosis, 9th ed: American College of Chest Physicians evidence-based clinical practice guidelines. Chest. 2012;141:e326S–e350S.

6. Gerbershagen HJ, Aduckathil S, van Wijck AJ, Peelen LM, Kalkman CJ, Meissner W. Pain intensity on the first day after surgery: a prospective cohort study comparing 179 surgical procedures. Anesthesiology. 2013; 118: 934-944.
7. Kehlet H, Dahl JB. The value of "multimodal" or "balanced analgesia" in postoperative pain treatment. Anesth Analg. 1993; 77: 1048-1056.
8. Marret E, Beloeil H, Lejus C. [What are the benefits and risk of non-opioid analgesics combined with postoperative opioids?]. Ann Fr Anesth Reanim. 2009; 28: e135-151.
9. Ménigaux C, Adam F, Guignard B, Sessler DI, Chauvin M. Preoperative gabapentin decreases anxiety and improves early functional recovery from knee surgery. Anesth Analg. 2005; 100: 1394-1399.
10. Sheen MJ, Ho ST, Lee CH, Tsung YC, Chang FL. Preoperative gabapentin prevents intrathecal morphine-induced pruritus after orthopedic surgery. Anesth Analg. 2008; 106: 1565-1872.
11. Fuzier R, Cuvillon P, Delcourt J, Lupescu R, Bonnemaison J, Bloc S, Theissen A. [Peripheral nerve block in orthopedic surgery: multicentric evaluation of practicing professionals and impact on the activity of the recovery room]. Ann Fr Anesth Reanim. 2007; 26: 761- 768.
12. Miller AG, McKenzie J, Greenky M, Shaw E, Gandhi K, Hozack WJ, Parvizi J. Spinal anesthesia: should everyone receive a urinary catheter?: a randomized, prospective study of patients undergoing total hip arthroplasty. *J Bone JointSurg Am* 2013; 95: 1498-1503 [PMID: 23965700 DOI: 10.2106/ JBJS.K.01671]
13. Chelly JE, Schilling D. Thromboprophylaxis and peripheral nerve blocks in patients undergoing joint arthroplasty. *J Arthroplasty* 2008; 23: 350-354 [PMID: 18358371 DOI: 10.1016/ j.arth.2007.05.045]
14. Brull R, McCartney CJ, Chan VW, El-Beheiry H. Neurological complications after regional anesthesia: contemporary estimates of risk. *Anesth Analg* 2007; 104: 965-974 [PMID: 17377115 DOI: 10.1213/01.ane.0000258740.17193.ec]
15. de Leeuw MA, Zuurmond WW, Perez RS. The psoas compartment block for hip surgery: the past, present, and future. *Anesthesiol Res Pract* 2011; 2011: 159541 [PMID: 21716721 DOI: 10.1155/2011/159541]
16. Fischer HB, Simanski CJ. A procedure-specific systematic review and consensus recommendations for analgesia after total hip replacement.

Anaesthesia 2005; 60: 1189-1202 [PMID: 16288617 DOI: 10.1111/j.1365-2044.2005.04382.x]

17. Luger TJ, Kammerlander C, Gosch M, Luger MF, Kammerlander-Knauer U, Roth T, Kreutziger J. Neuroaxial versus general anesthesia in geriatric patients for hip fracture surgery: does it matter? *Osteoporos Int* 2010; 21: S555-S572[PMID: 21057995 DOI: 10.1007/s00198-010-1399-7]

18. Hu F, Jiang C, Shen J, Tang P, Wang Y. Preoperativepredictors for mortality following hip fracture surgery: a systematic review and meta-analysis. *Injury* 2012; 43: 676-685 [PMID: 21683355 DOI: 10.1016/j.injury.2011.05.017]

19. Modig J. Regional anesthesia and blood loss. *Acta AnaesthesiolScand Suppl* 1988; 89: 44-48 [PMID: 3067490 DOI:10.1111/j.1399-6576.1988.tb02842.x]

20. Borghi B, Casati A, Iuorio S, Celleno D, Michael M, Serafini P, Pusceddu A, Fanelli G. Frequency of hypotension and bradycardia during general anesthesia, epidural anesthesia,or integrated epidural-general anesthesia for total hip replacement. *J Clin Anesth* 2002; 14: 102-106 [PMID: 11943521 DOI: 10.1016/s0952-8180(01)00362-2]

21. Neuman MD, Silber JH, Elkassabany NM, Ludwig JM, Fleisher LA. Comparative effectiveness of regional versus general anesthesia for hip fracture surgery in adults. *Anesthesiology* 2012; 117: 72-92 [PMID: 22713634 DOI: 10.1097/ALN.0b013e3182545e7c]

22. Regan EA, Radcliff TA, Henderson WG, Cowper Ripley DC, Maciejewski ML, Vogel WB, Hutt E. Improving hip fractures outcomes for COPD patients. *COPD* 2013; 10: 11-19 [PMID: 23272668 DOI: 10.3109/15412555.2012.723072]

23. Stafford-Smith M. Impaired haemostasis and regional anesthesia. Can J Anaesth. 1996;43:R129–R141.

24. Donaldson J, Thomson HE, Harper NJ, Kenny NW. Bone cement implantation syndrome. Br J Anaesth 2009; 102: 12–22

25. Sasano N, Ishida S, Tetsu S, et al. Cerebral fat embolism diagnosed by magnetic resonance imaging at one, eight and 50 days after hip arthroplasty: a case report. Can J Anaesth 2004; 51:875–9.

SURGICAL APPROACH

SURGICAL APPROACH: MODIFIED DIRECT LATERAL APPROACH

Exposure of the hip joint through partial release of interial fibers of vastus lateralis and gluteus medius muscles from greater trochanter is popularly called as direct lateral approach of hip.

This approach was first described by McFarland and Osborne (1954). The method was mainly centered with a thought of preserving the integrity of gluteus medius muscle. They recognized that gluteus medius and vastus lateralis are in direct functional continuity through tendinous periosteum that span greater trochanter. A single flap consisting of gluteus medius and vastus lateralis was detached from greater trochantor and taken forward which was sutured back in place.

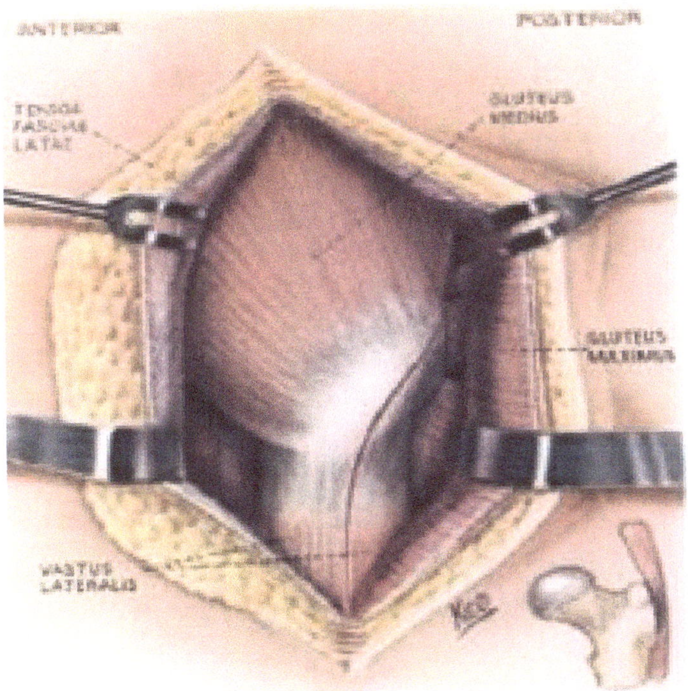

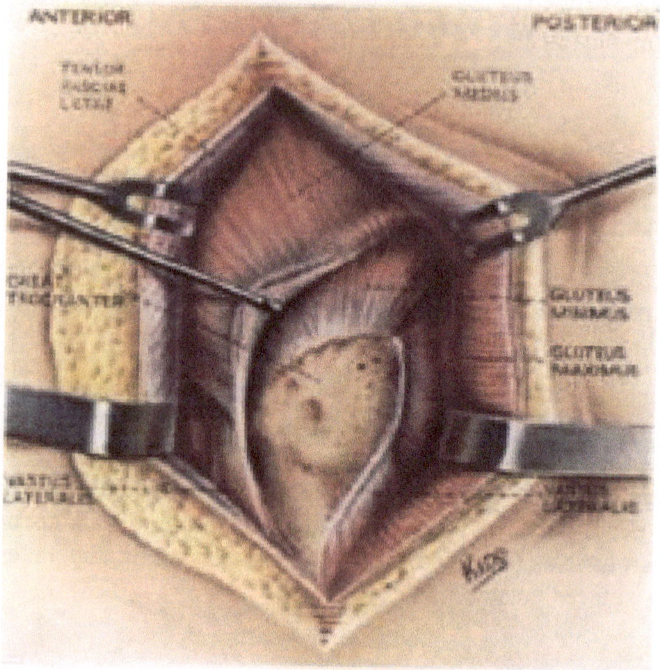

Line of incision is at posterior margin of gluteus medius with anterior displacement of gluteus medius and vastus lateralis in continuity.

In 1982, Kevin hardinge came with an idea of preserving main bulk of gluteus medius by detaiching only its anterior fibers. This approach allowed the patients to be place in supine position which according to hardinge offered optimal condition for orientation of implant and correction of limb length.

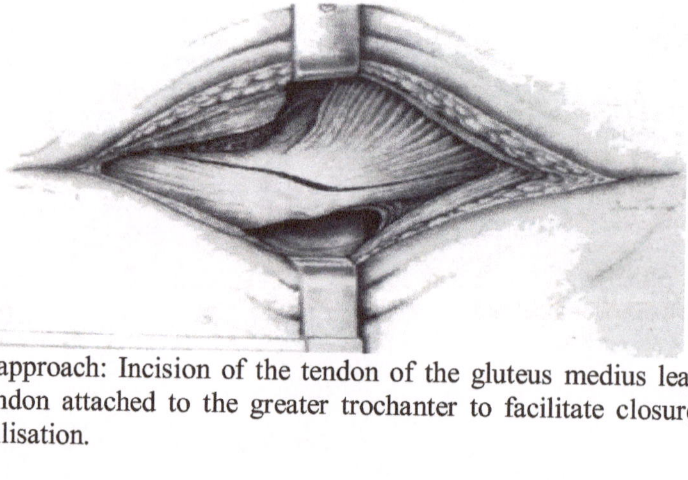

Hardinge approach: Incision of the tendon of the gluteus medius leaves a cuff of tendon attached to the greater trochanter to facilitate closure and early mobilisation.

V.S Pai In 2002 from new zealand modified some of the concept of hardinge approach. He advocated using direct lateral approach for hemiarhtroplasty and total hip replacement. Patient was place in full lateral position with skin incision made between anterior and posterior borders of greater trochanter then divided gluteus medius between anterior 1/3rd and posterior 2/3rd using electric cautery and sharp dissection. A flap was elevated consisting of anterior part of gluteus medius and vastus lateralis leaving behind posterior bulk of gluteus medius intact.

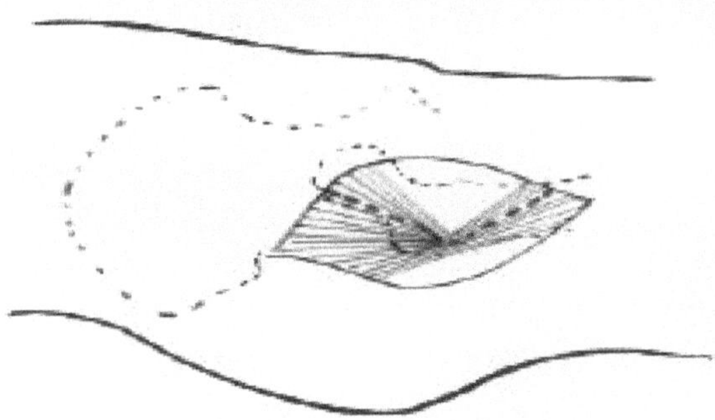

Modified harding approach: Abductor split is made between anterior one-third and posterior two-third of the gluteus medius.

Our approach:

Pre op radiograph: pelvis with both hip joint with traction and 15 degree internal rotation.

Positioning:

After spinal epidural anesthesia, patient is placed in lateral positions with involved side facing upward and side support is applied.

After scrubbing painting and draping, sterile hip drape is raped over the patients.

Incision: (Our Approach)

Feel for the greater trochanter anterior and posterior border and mark the greater trochanter tip. The incision is made mid way between anterior and posterior border of greater trochanter centerd over its tip.

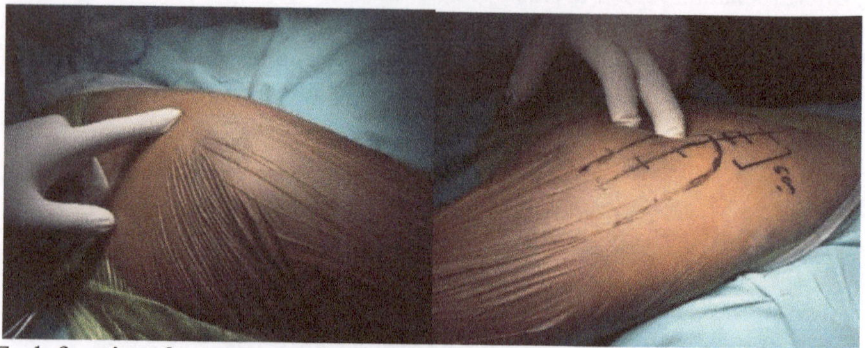

Feel for tip of greater trochanter and marking of anterior and posterior border. Incision made midway between both the borders not extending beyond 5cm from tip of greater trochanter. Superiarly (cephalic direction).

Deep Dissection:

After skin and subcutaneous tissue is incised and retracted, tensor fascia lata is indentified and split in line with the skin incision and charnely self retaining retractor is applied.

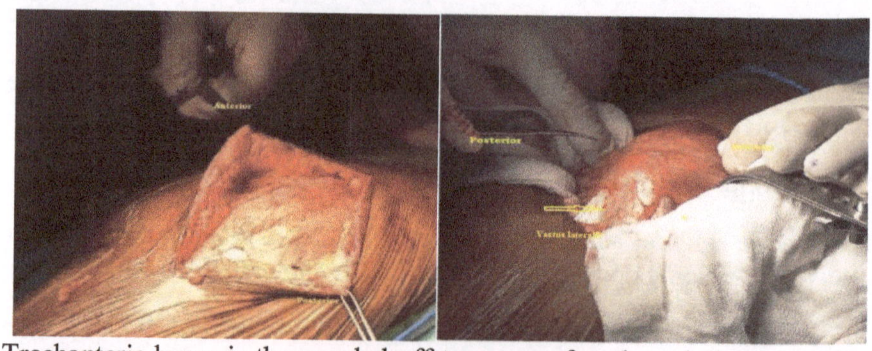

Trochanteric busra is then peeled off to expose fan shaped gluteus medius and vastus lateralis. Greater trochanter lies in the centre of the incision, and the gluteus medius is identified by its crescent shaped insertion on greater trochanter which is divided into its **anterior two third and posterior one third.**

Note *:Splitting of gluteus medius at junction of ant two third and post one third is a modification by us contrary to the conventional lateral approach where the surgeons split the gluteus at junction of ant one third and post two third.*

This is based on the fact that the post 3rd of gluteus medius fibers attaching over tip of GT are sufficiently strong abductors, more so the flap is elevated with a chip of bone from GT which once sutured back gives good bone to bone healing and leaving no chance of any abductor weakness. Moreover elevating ant 2rd of gluteus medius gives better viewof proximal femur and makes it easy to prepare canal

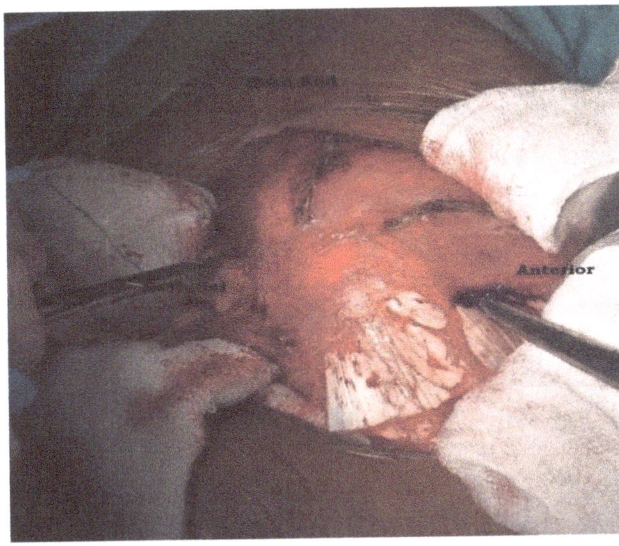

With the help of electric cautery the line of incision is marked. An osteoperiosteal sliver of bone from greator trochanter is osteotomised with a curved osteotome .And thus flap consisting of tendons of vastus lateralis and gluteus medius in continuety is reflected anteriorly.

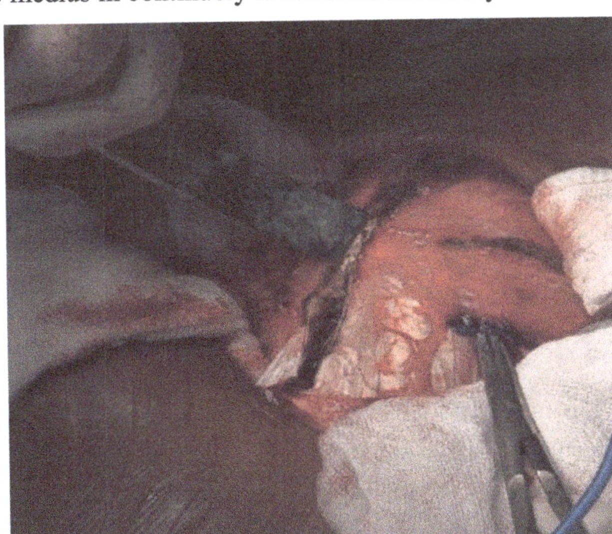

Thin chip of bone is chiselled along with fibers of anterior 2/3rd of gluteus medius and vastus lateralis.

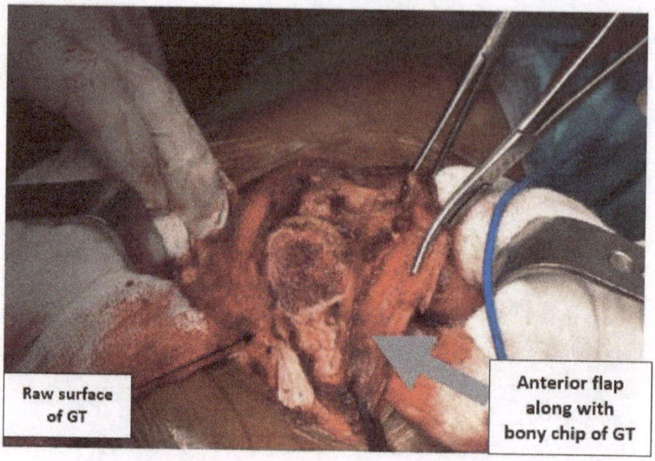

The incision is extended distally over the lateral aspects greater trochanter thus dividing the vastus lateralis. With the help of cautery anterior capsules of hip is exposed by gradually externally rotating the limb and elevating the anterior muscle falp. The medial border of proximal femur is exposed from calcar to lesser trochanter. "T" shaped incision is made on anterior capsules (which is mostly torn in case of trauma) to expose the head. The head is now delivered using bone lever or corkscrew.

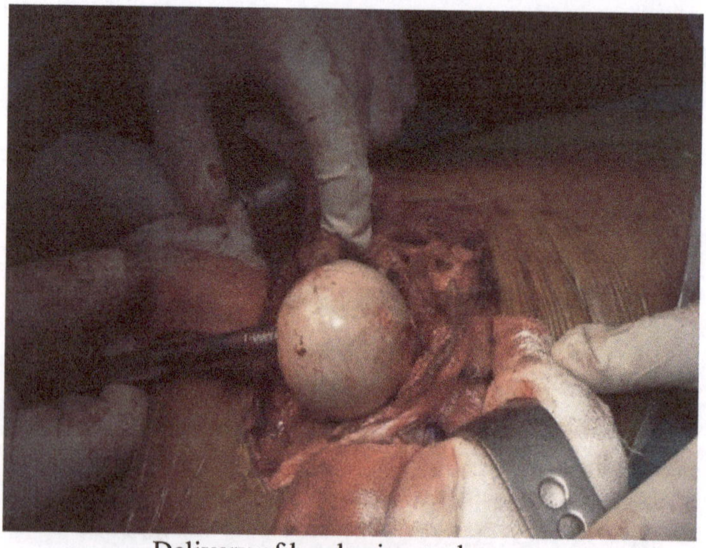

Delivery of head using corkscrew.

Preparation of femur:

After delivering head, leg is held perpendicular to the floor and then externally rotated in figure of 4 manner. Now neck is trimmed leaving one finger breadth of calcar preserved on which the implant will sit.

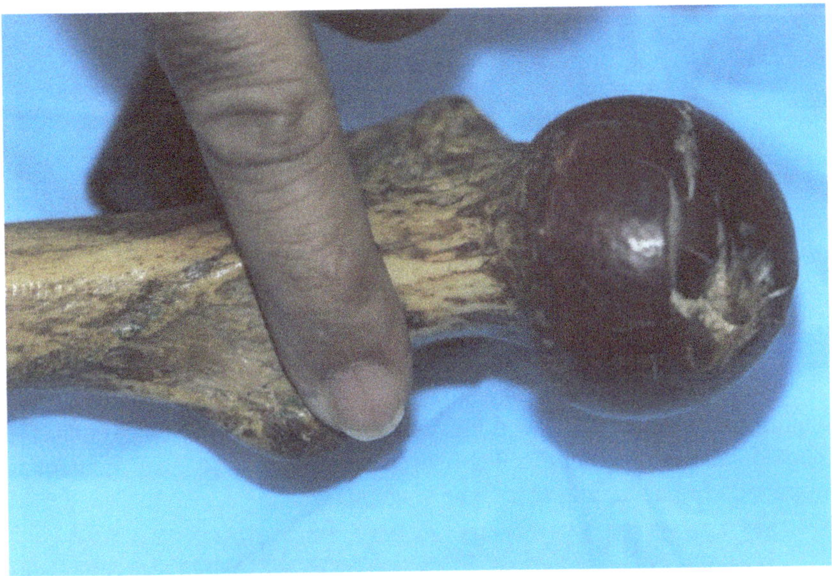

Trimming of neck leaving one finger breadth of calcar preserved.

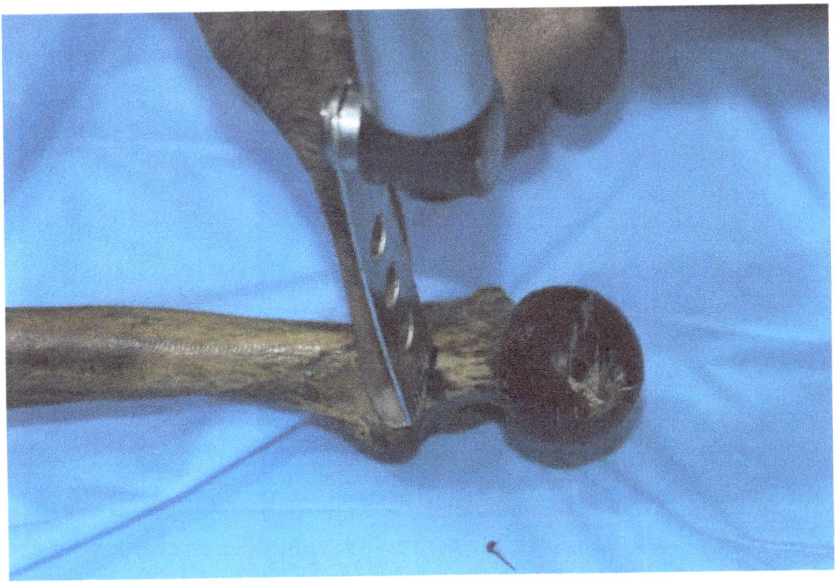

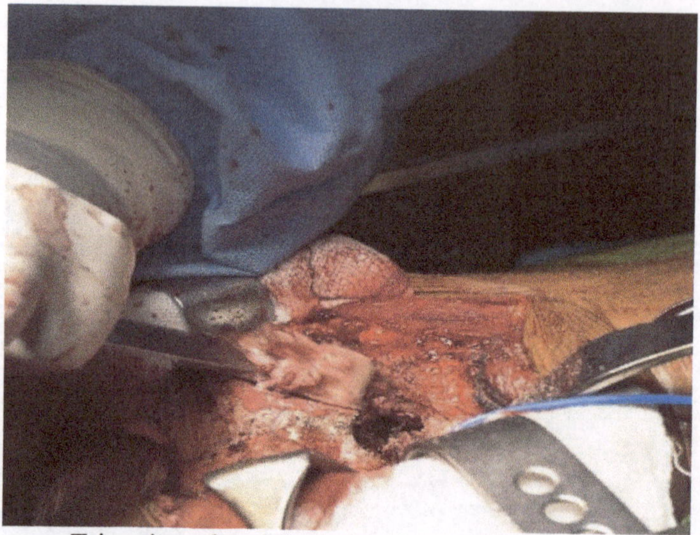

Trimming of neck is done using oscillating saw.

Broaching of femur is now done using different types of broaches for cemented and un-cemented stems. We preferred to use cement for osteoporotic femur having Dorr type C canal.

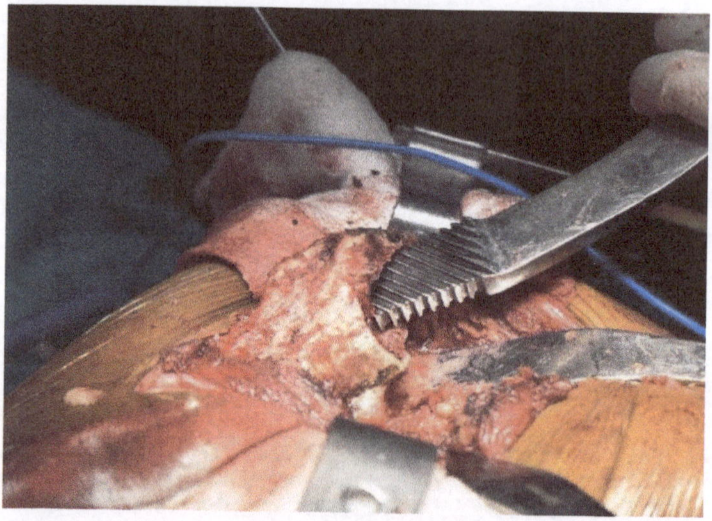

Preparation of femur.

While broaching the version should be kept in mind. We prefer lesser trochanter as a land mark for intra op version control. Lesser trochanter has been found to correlate with posterior condylar axis of femur which can serve a good land mark for intra op version control.

Now head is measured for its size. We have head size ranging from 37 to 55 mm with 1m increments which prevents use of inappropriate head size and subsequently early failure of the prosthesis.

Note :*A head of inadequate size can exert an Hertizan effect leading to early implant failure. In most part of the world surgeons prefer to put smaller size head if exact size not available, but as can be seen in chapter of mathematical calculation, a smaller head has greater adverse effect on acetabulum then a larger head thus unlike many surgeons we preffer a size larger head if exact size is unavailable*

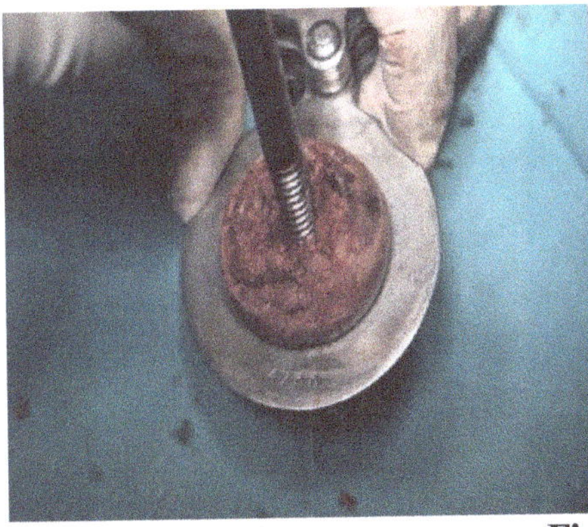

Figure-1.

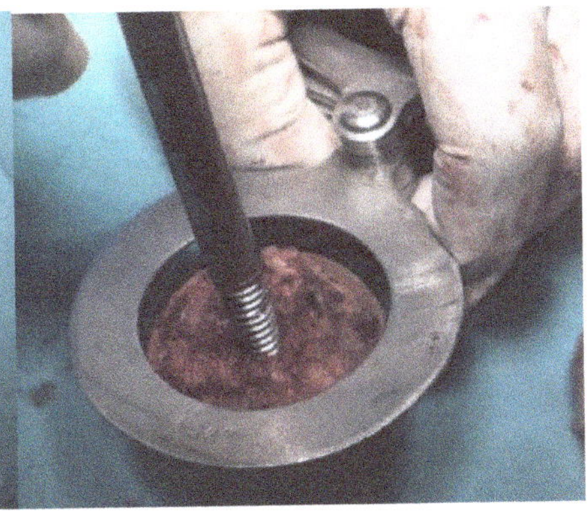

Figure-2.

The extracted head is not passing thru head sizer of 47mm (Fig.1) and just passes through 48mm sizer. (fig-2) We chose head size of 48mm rather 47mm for this patient.

Note-The common surgical practice, to use one size smaller head dimetter of the prosthethis than what is extracted from the patients during surgery we want to emphasize that it is incorrect and gives hertzian contact stress (mathematical culculation) and which is very detrimental for long term survival of the prosthethis.

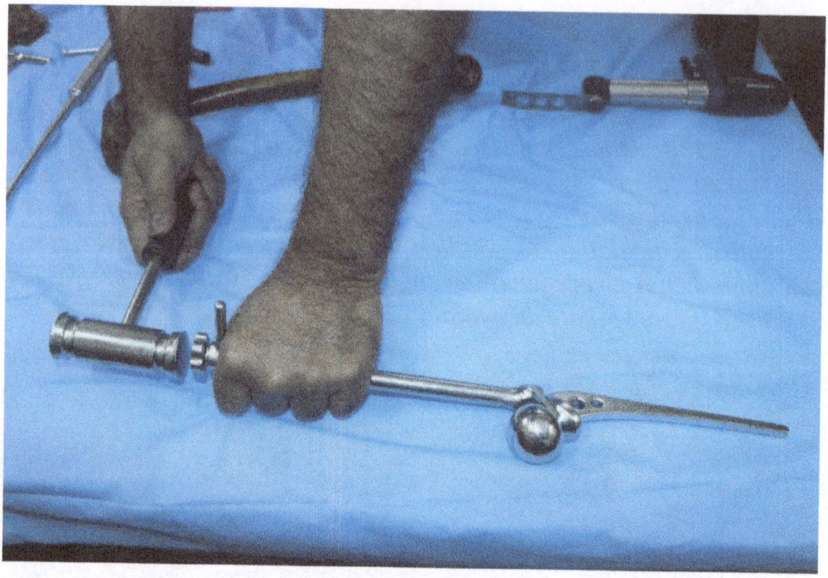

Femoral stem holder and version guide with hammering attachment.

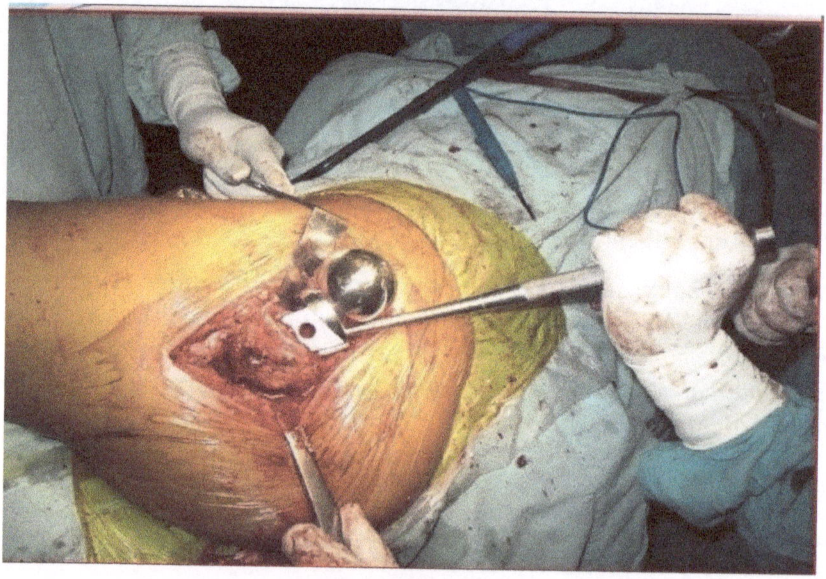

Where to hammer.

- **<u>Criteria to move to *Phase IV:*</u>** 4+/5 of all LE musculature, minimal to no pain or swelling

Phase IV: Advanced Strengthening and Higher Level Functioning

- **<u>Goals:</u>** Return to appropriate sports/recreational activities, enhance strength, endurance, and proprioception
- **<u>Exercises:</u>** Progress above exercises, increase duration of endurance activities, return-to-work tasks, squatting
- **<u>Criteria for discharge:</u>** Non antalgic and independent gait, independent in step over step stair climbing, pain-free AROM, 4+/5 LE strength, normal age-appropriate balance and proprioception, and independent in home exercise program

REFFERENCES

1. Hardinge K. The direct lateral approach to the hip. J Bone Joint Surg Br. 1982;64:17–9.
2. Singh JA. Epidemiology of knee and hip arthroplasty: A systematic review. Open Orthop J. 2011;5:80–5
3. McFarland B, Osborne G. Approach to the hip: A suggested improvement on Kocher's method. J Bone Joint Surg Br. 1954;36B:364–7.
4. Smith-Petersen MN. Approach to and exposure of the hip joint for mold arthroplasty. J Bone Joint Surg Am. 1949;31A:40–6.
5. Restrepo C, Parvizi J, Pour AE, Hozack WJ. Prospective randomized study of two surgical approaches for total hip arthroplasty. J Arthroplasty. 2010;25:671–9.el
6. Barrett WP, Turner SE, Leopold JP. Prospective randomized study of direct anterior vs. postero-lateral approach for total hip arthroplasty. J Arthroplasty. 2013;28:1634–8.
7. Witzleb WC, Stephan L, Krummenauer F, Neuke A, Günther KP. Short-term outcome after posterior versus lateral surgical approach for total hip arthroplasty – A randomized clinical trial. Eur J Med Res. 2009;14:256–63
8. Martin CT, Pugely AJ, Gao Y, Clark CR. A comparison of hospital length of stay and short-term morbidity between the anterior and the posterior approaches to total hip arthroplasty. J Arthroplasty. 2013;28:849–54.

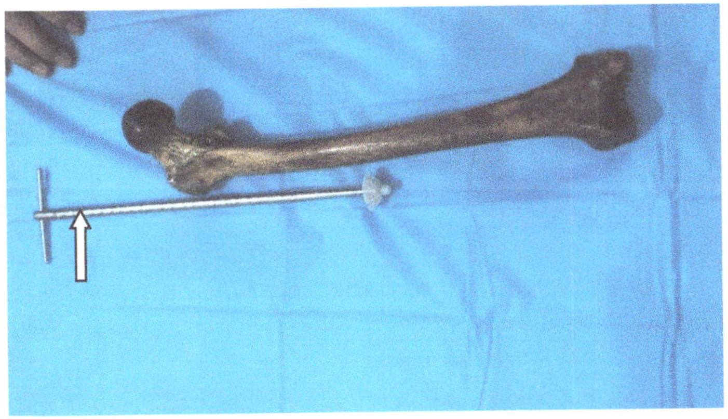

Note-18cm from the tip of the GT restrictor can be place (not mandatory) Provides equal limb length, correct offset, and thus prolongs survival of the system (minimum 21 years till date).

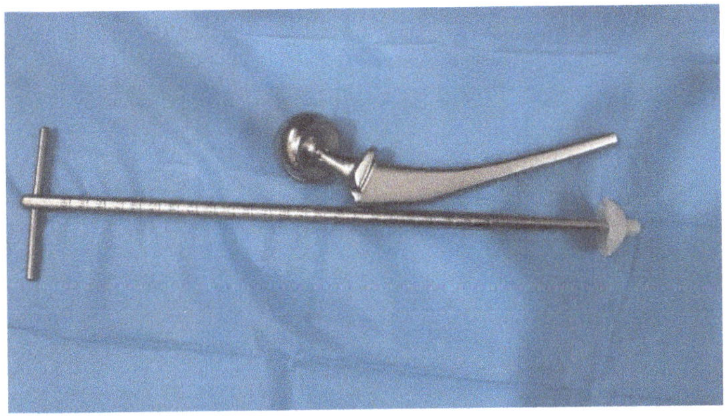

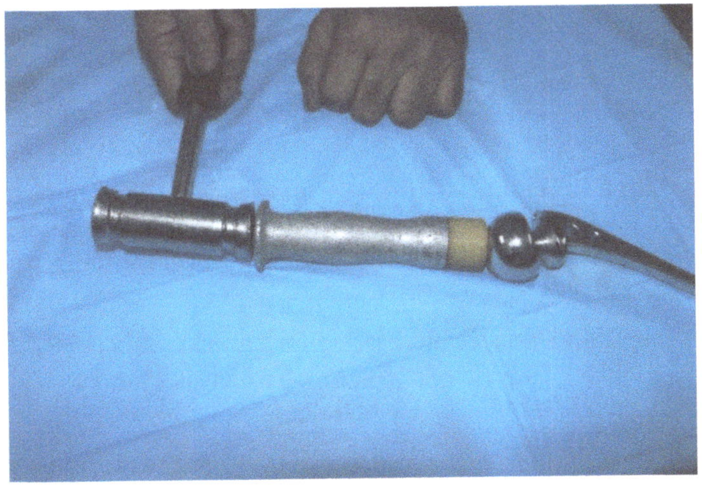

Wrong practise (contra indicated).

Appropriate size of prosthesis thus chosen is introduced in the femur. It is necessary to give the femoral component correct anti-version which is necessary for longevity of the implant. Generally 15 degree of femoral anti-version is given we use lesser trochanter as guide for correct version the anterior border of lesser trochanter should be collinear with posterior border of the collar prosthesis.

Note : It was because of our extensive work on cadavers with the aluminium model of prosthesis that we get to know that if the posterior border of the collar of prosthesis coincides with the anterior margin of lesser trochanter we almost get an anatomical version.

The head of prosthesis is relocated in to the acetabulum and stability of joint is checked for various moments. Now closer is started in layers with no.1 vicryl starting with anterior capsular repair if possible to attachment of gluteus medius to greater trochanter with the help of osteotendinous suturing.

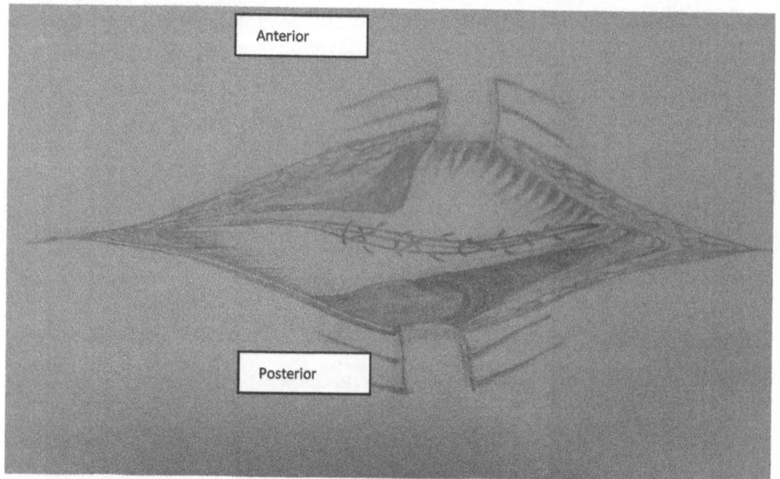

Suturing of glutius medius to greater trochanter.

Post Operative Protocol- patients were allowed to sit from the next day of surgery with back support, and were made to stand after change of dressing and Foleys was taken out after 48 hrs of surgery also the drain were taken out at the same time .

Patients were kept on non weight bearing for 2 weeks and partial wt bearing was allowed for another 2 weeks following which full weight bearing was allowed with help of zimmer frame walking.

Physiotherapy with on bed knee and hip ROM were started immediate post op and were continued in asset pattern which is common in almost all kind of hip replacement and is as described below

Phase I: Immediately Post-Operatively (Days 0-3)

- **Goals:** Perform bed mobility and transfers with minimal assistance while maintaining WB precautions, ambulate 25-100 feet w/ assistive device, stair training as appropriate for home ambulation, independently perform SLR, regain 80° PROM and AROM flexion, verbalize precautions
- **Exercises:** Quad, hamstring, and glute sets, gait training on levelsurfaces, PROM exercises, SLRs, soft tissue massage, transfer training
- **Modalities:** Cryotherapy application 5 times daily and 20 min before/after exercise program
- **Precautions:** WBAT w/ assistive device, monitor wound healing and signs for DVT and PE, no exercises with weights or resistance, avoid torque and twisting forces across knee
- **Criteria to move to *Phase II:*** AROM: Hip flexion 0-90°, hip abduction 0-30°, independent in transfers and ambulation for 100 feet w/ assistive device

Phase II: Motion Phase (Day 3-Week 6)

- **Goals:** Muscle strengthening of entire hip girdle, begin proprioceptive training, continue with gait, endurance, and functional training and mobility
- **Exercises:**
  - **Weeks 1-4:** AROM hip abduction, quad, hamstring, and glut isometrics, heelslides, gait training, stationary biking, closed chai proprioception exercises
  - **Weeks 4-6:** Continue/progress above exercises with resistance tolerated, front/lateral step up/downs, ¼ front lunge, sit to sta exercises, ambulation on uneven surfaces
- **Criteria to move to *Phase III:*** AROM of hip motion 0-110°, go quad control, independently ambulates 800 feet w/o assistive device gait deviations

Phase III: Intermediate Phase (Weeks 7-12)

- **Goals:** Adequate strength of all LE musculature, return to n functional activities
- **Exercises:** Progress with above strengthening, endurance, proprioception exercises

9. Malek IA, Royce G, Bhatti SU, Whittaker JP, Phillips SP, Wilson IR, et al. A comparison between the direct anterior and posterior approaches for total hip arthroplasty: The role of an 'Enhanced Recovery' pathway. Bone Joint J. 2016;98-B:754–60

10. Sheth D, Cafri G, Inacio MC, Paxton EW, Namba RS. Anterior and anterolateral approaches for THA are associated with lower dislocation risk without higher revision risk. Clin Orthop Relat Res. 2015;473:3401–8.

11. Mulliken BD, Rorabeck CH, Bourne RB, Nayak N. A modified direct lateral approach in total hip arthroplasty: A comprehensive review. J Arthroplasty. 1998;13:737–47.

12. Demos HA, Rorabeck CH, Bourne RB, MacDonald SJ, McCalden RW. Instability in primary total hip arthroplasty with the direct lateral approach. Clin Orthop Relat Res. 2001;393:168–80.

13. Kenin GS. Parker, MJ. Hemiarthroplasty of the hip. The anterior or the posterior approach. A comparison of surgical approaches. Injury 1993 24 9. 611- 613

DESIGNER CHANGES

The abductor musculature, acting on a lever arm extending form the lateral aspect of the greater trochanter to the center of the femoral head, must exert an equal moment to hold the pelvis level when in one-legged stance and a greater moment to tilt the pelvis on to the same side when walking or running. Since the ratio of the length of the lever arm to the body weight to that of the abductor musculature is about **2.5:1**, the force of the abductor muscles must approximate 2.5 times the body weight to maintain the pelvis level when standing on one leg.

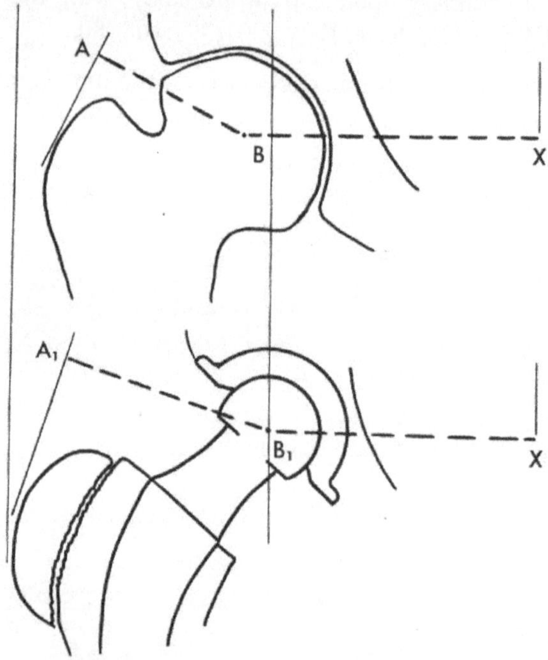

The forces on the joint act not only in the coronal plane, but because the body's center of gravity (in the midline anterior to the second sacral vertebral body) is posterior to the axis of the joint, they also act in the sagittal plane to bend the stem posteriorly.

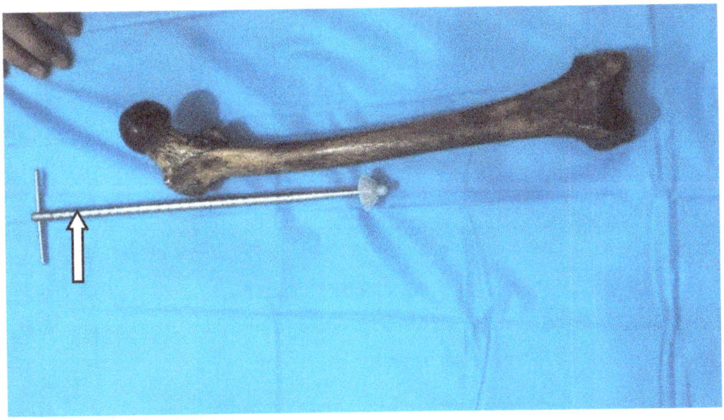

Note-18cm from the tip of the GT restrictor can be place (not mandatory) Provides equal limb length, correct offset, and thus prolongs survival of the system (minimum 21 years till date).

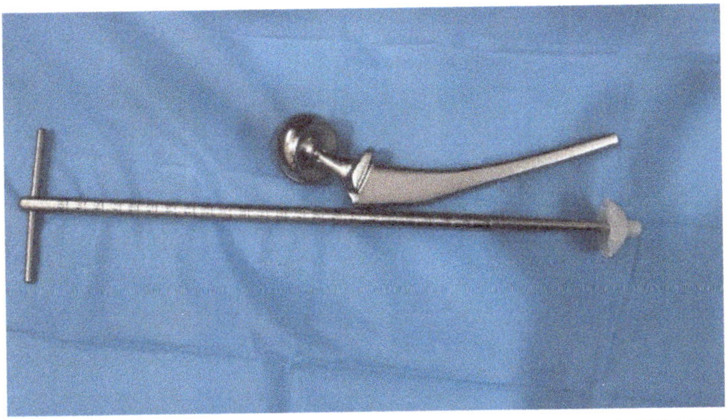

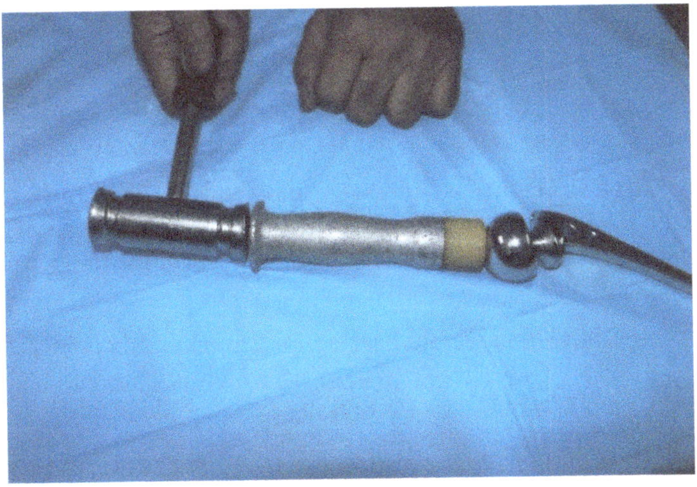

Wrong practise (contra indicated).

Appropriate size of prosthesis thus chosen is introduced in the femur. It is necessary to give the femoral component correct anti-version which is necessary for longevity of the implant. Generally 15 degree of femoral anti-version is given we use lesser trochanter as guide for correct version the anterior border of lesser trochanter should be collinear with posterior border of the collar prosthesis.

***Note** : It was because of our extensive work on cadavers with the aluminium model of prosthesis that we get to know that if the posterior border of the collar of prosthesis coincides with the anterior margin of lesser trochanter we almost get an anatomical version.*

The head of prosthesis is relocated in to the acetabulum and stability of joint is checked for various moments. Now closer is started in layers with no.1 vicryl starting with anterior capsular repair if possible to attachment of gluteus medius to greater trochanter with the help of osteotendinous suturing.

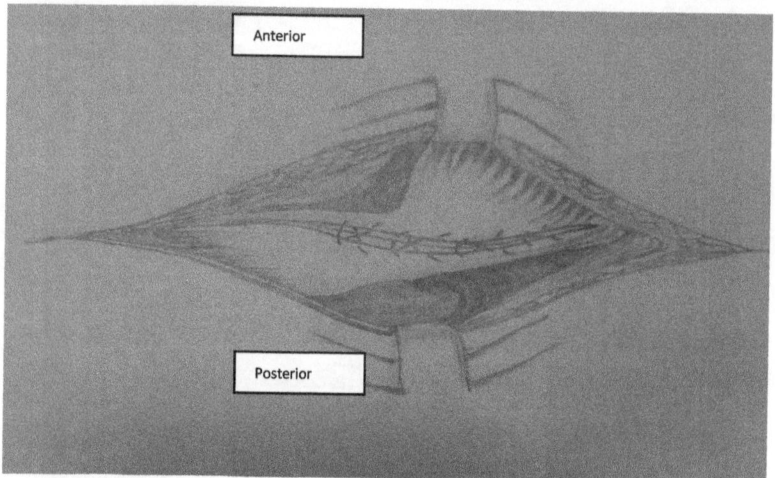

Suturing of glutius medius to greater trochanter.

Post Operative Protocol- patients were allowed to sit from the next day of surgery with back support, and were made to stand after change of dressing and Foleys was taken out after 48 hrs of surgery also the drain were taken out at the same time .

Patients were kept on non weight bearing for 2 weeks and partial wt bearing was allowed for another 2 weeks following which full weight bearing was allowed with help of zimmer frame walking.

Physiotherapy with on bed knee and hip ROM were started immediate post op and were continued in asset pattern which is common in almost all kind of hip replacement and is as described below

Phase I: Immediately Post-Operatively (Days 0-3)

- **Goals:** Perform bed mobility and transfers with minimal assistance while maintaining WB precautions, ambulate 25-100 feet w/ assistive device, stair training as appropriate for home ambulation, independently perform SLR, regain 80° PROM and AROM flexion, verbalize precautions
- **Exercises:** Quad, hamstring, and glute sets, gait training on levelsurfaces, PROM exercises, SLRs, soft tissue massage, transfer training
- **Modalities:** Cryotherapy application 5 times daily and 20 min before/after exercise program
- **Precautions:** WBAT w/ assistive device, monitor wound healing and signs for DVT and PE, no exercises with weights or resistance, avoid torque and twisting forces across knee
- **Criteria to move to *Phase II:*** AROM: Hip flexion 0-90°, hip abduction 0-30°, independent in transfers and ambulation for 100 feet w/ assistive device

Phase II: Motion Phase (Day 3-Week 6)

- **Goals:** Muscle strengthening of entire hip girdle, begin proprioceptive training, continue with gait, endurance, and functional training and mobility
- **Exercises:**
    - **Weeks 1-4:** AROM hip abduction, quad, hamstring, and glute isometrics, heelslides, gait training, stationary biking, closed chain proprioception exercises
    - **Weeks 4-6:** Continue/progress above exercises with resistance as tolerated, front/lateral step up/downs, ¼ front lunge, sit to stand exercises, ambulation on uneven surfaces
- **Criteria to move to *Phase III:*** AROM of hip motion 0-110°, good quad control, independently ambulates 800 feet w/o assistive device or gait deviations

Phase III: Intermediate Phase (Weeks 7-12)

- **Goals:** Adequate strength of all LE musculature, return to most functional activities
- **Exercises:** Progress with above strengthening, endurance, and proprioception exercises

- **Criteria to move to *Phase IV:*** 4+/5 of all LE musculature, minimal to no pain or swelling

Phase IV: Advanced Strengthening and Higher Level Functioning

- **Goals:** Return to appropriate sports/recreational activities, enhance strength, endurance, and proprioception
- **Exercises:** Progress above exercises, increase duration of endurance activities, return-to-work tasks, squatting
- **Criteria for discharge:** Non antalgic and independent gait, independent in step over step stair climbing, pain-free AROM, 4+/5 LE strength, normal age-appropriate balance and proprioception, and independent in home exercise program

REFFERENCES

1. Hardinge K. The direct lateral approach to the hip. J Bone Joint Surg Br. 1982;64:17–9.
2. Singh JA. Epidemiology of knee and hip arthroplasty: A systematic review. Open Orthop J. 2011;5:80–5
3. McFarland B, Osborne G. Approach to the hip: A suggested improvement on Kocher's method. J Bone Joint Surg Br. 1954;36B:364–7.
4. Smith-Petersen MN. Approach to and exposure of the hip joint for mold arthroplasty. J Bone Joint Surg Am. 1949;31A:40–6.
5. Restrepo C, Parvizi J, Pour AE, Hozack WJ. Prospective randomized study of two surgical approaches for total hip arthroplasty. J Arthroplasty. 2010;25:671–9.e1
6. Barrett WP, Turner SE, Leopold JP. Prospective randomized study of direct anterior vs. postero-lateral approach for total hip arthroplasty. J Arthroplasty. 2013;28:1634–8.
7. Witzleb WC, Stephan L, Krummenauer F, Neuke A, Günther KP. Short-term outcome after posterior versus lateral surgical approach for total hip arthroplasty – A randomized clinical trial. Eur J Med Res. 2009;14:256–63
8. Martin CT, Pugely AJ, Gao Y, Clark CR. A comparison of hospital length of stay and short-term morbidity between the anterior and the posterior approaches to total hip arthroplasty. J Arthroplasty. 2013;28:849–54.

9. Malek IA, Royce G, Bhatti SU, Whittaker JP, Phillips SP, Wilson IR, et al. A comparison between the direct anterior and posterior approaches for total hip arthroplasty: The role of an 'Enhanced Recovery' pathway. Bone Joint J. 2016;98-B:754–60

10. Sheth D, Cafri G, Inacio MC, Paxton EW, Namba RS. Anterior and anterolateral approaches for THA are associated with lower dislocation risk without higher revision risk. Clin Orthop Relat Res. 2015;473:3401–8.

11. Mulliken BD, Rorabeck CH, Bourne RB, Nayak N. A modified direct lateral approach in total hip arthroplasty: A comprehensive review. J Arthroplasty. 1998;13:737–47.

12. Demos HA, Rorabeck CH, Bourne RB, MacDonald SJ, McCalden RW. Instability in primary total hip arthroplasty with the direct lateral approach. Clin Orthop Relat Res. 2001;393:168–80.

13. Kenin GS. Parker, MJ. Hemiarthroplasty of the hip. The anterior or the posterior approach. A comparison of surgical approaches. Injury 1993 24 9. 611- 613

DESIGNER CHANGES

The abductor musculature, acting on a lever arm extending form the lateral aspect of the greater trochanter to the center of the femoral head, must exert an equal moment to hold the pelvis level when in one-legged stance and a greater moment to tilt the pelvis on to the same side when walking or running. Since the ratio of the length of the lever arm to the body weight to that of the abductor musculature is about **2.5:1**, the force of the abductor muscles must approximate 2.5 times the body weight to maintain the pelvis level when standing on one leg.

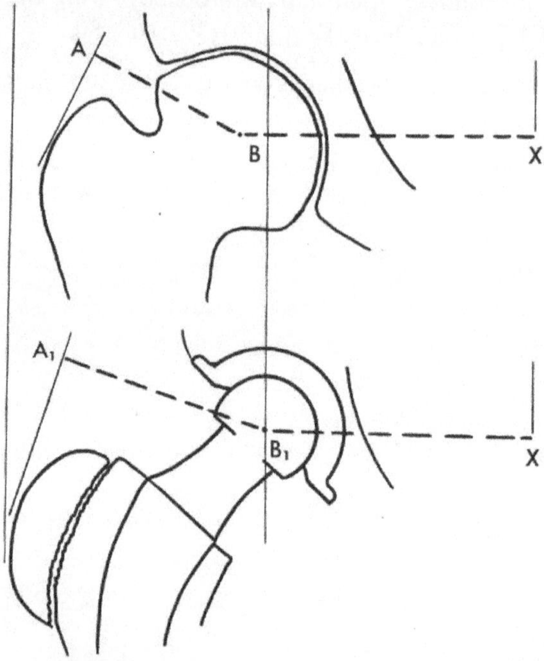

The forces on the joint act not only in the coronal plane, but because the body's center of gravity (in the midline anterior to the second sacral vertebral body) is posterior to the axis of the joint, they also act in the sagittal plane to bend the stem posteriorly.

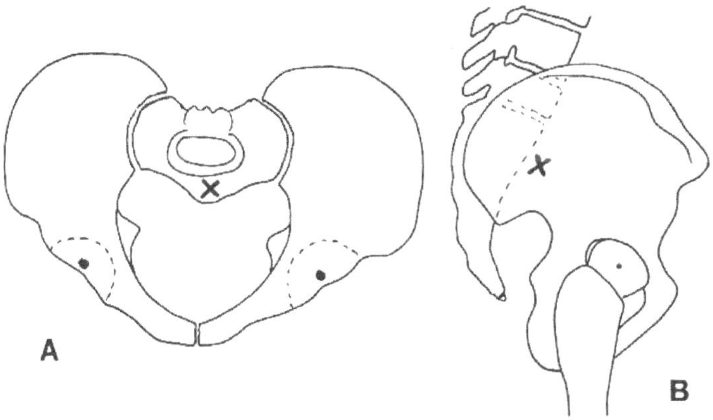

The forces acting in this direction are increased when the loaded hip is flexed, as when arising form a chair, ascending or descending stairs on an incline, or lifting.

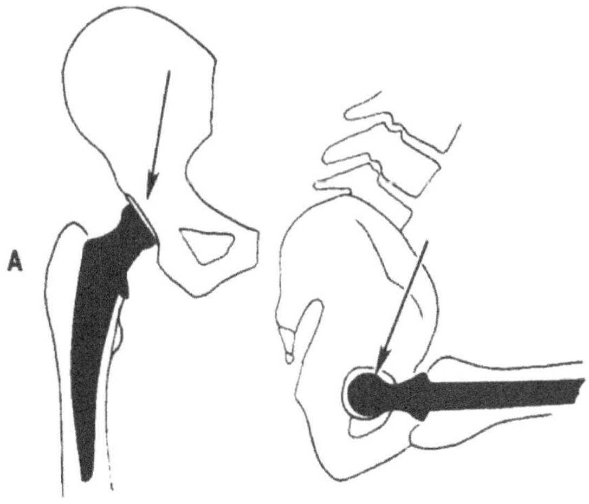

Such forces cause posterior deflection or retroversion of the femoral component.

Rotational stability of the stem can be increased both proximally and distally. Increasing the **width of the proximal portion of the stem** to better fill the metaphysis increases the torsional stability of femoral component, especially when it is implanted without cement. Freemanfound that the fracture rotational stability of both cemented and cementless femoral components also can be improved substantially by retention of a longer segment of the femoral neck, therefore the importance of the calcar. Modification of the distal portion of the stem may add to rotational stability as well. **A rounded, rectangular cross-section** resists rotation within a cement mantle better than a circular one.

The ideal femoral reconstruction produces a normal center of rotation of the femoral head. This location is determined by three factors:

i. Vertical height (vertical offset)
ii. Medial offset (horizontal offset)
iii. Version of the femoral neck (anterior offset)

Medial offset is the distance from the center of the femoral head to a line through the axis of the distal part of the stem. Inadequate restoration of this offset shortens the moment arm of the abductor musculature and results in increased joint reaction force, limp and body impingement, which may result in dislocation. Conversely, an excessive increases in offset results in increased stresses within the stem and cement mantle that may lead is stem fracture or loosening.

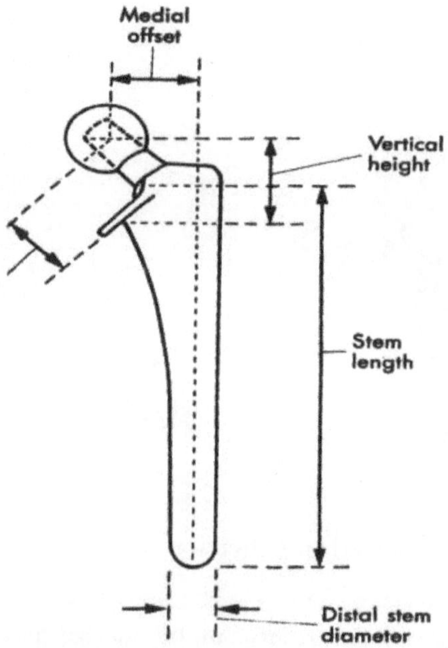

If a prosthesis with a small femoral head is used, the diameter of the neck approaches close to that of the head to keep the neck strong enough, and the neck tends to impinge on the edge of the cup even in a shorter arc of motion.

Therefore, the socket's depth and beveled edges and the greater diameter of the head in comparison to the neck in hip prosthesis with larger heads are features that allow a greater range of motion.

The **coefficient of friction** in normal joints has been estimated as 0.008 to 0.02. Walker and Bullough estimated the coefficient of friction of metal-on-metal joints tested in vivo as approximately 0.8 and that of metal on high-density polyethylene as approximately 0.02. A frictional torque is produced when the loaded hip moves through an arc of motion. It is the product of the friction force times the length of the lever arm that is, the distance a given point on surface or the head moves during a given arc of motion.

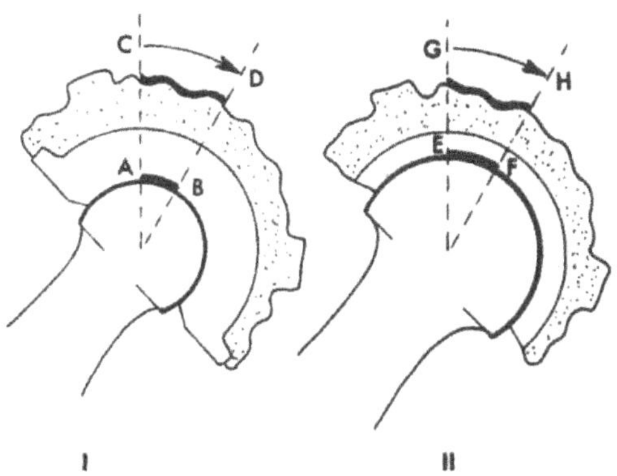

Frictional force depends on the coefficient of friction, the applied load, and the surface area of contact between the head and the socket.

This frictional torque is transmitted to the cup, the stem of the femoral component, the surrounding cement and the cement bone interface or directly on the stem - bone interface as a force that tends to twist the component.

The decreased frictional torque force created by a smaller head is the reason Charnley chose a **22mm diameter head** and referred to his metal-on-polyethylene procedure as a low frictional torque arthroplasty. Morrey and Ilstrupdemonstrated a higher incidence of acetabular lossening with a 32mm head than with the original 22mm Charnley component.

Wear can be defined as the loss of material from the surfaces of the prosthesis as a result of motion between those surfaces. A low coefficient of friction does not necessary correlate with good wear characteristics. Charnley estimated that high-density polyethylene is at least 16.5 times more durable than Teflon which has a very low coefficient of friction. Wear is difficult to measure accurately. **Bragdon, O'Connor and Lowenstein** designed a hip simulator that more closely initiates human hip motion.

Clinical roentgenographic studies usually report linear wear rates, whereas in vitro studies often report volumetric wear.Nashed, Becker and Gustilofound a wear rate of 0.25mm a year when a titanium head was coupled with a cementless, metal backed acetabular component. Bono, Sanford, and Toussaint reported average wear of 0.77mm a year in a group of patients with early failure of a cementless acetabular component that used a nonhemispherical liner with excessively thin polyethylene in high stress areas at the periphery of the implant. The physical properties of polyethylene also affect its rate of wear. Molecular weight has been correlated with the wear resistance of polyethylene. The biological consequences of particular wear debris are cause for concern; birefringement particles consistent with polyethylene debris are routinely identified in the membranes surrounding failed total hip replacements.

Stress transfer to the femur is desirable because it provides a physiological stimulus for maintaining bone mass and preventing disuse osteoporosis.

Using video densitometry analysis of autopsy retrieved femur, Maloney et al found that both cemented and uncemented implants, the area of greatest decrease in bone mineral density occurred in the proximal medial cortex. If a prosthesis has a collar that seated on the cut surface of the neck, it is postulated that axial loading of the bone will occur in this area.

There has been variable results in various studies regarding longevity of bipolar prosthesis ,where different design of bipolar have been used suggesting that it is a design based phenomenon as well, this and the understanding of desired biomechanical performance by a prosthesis as explained above has lead to evolution of the BHU Bipolar prosthesis.

The science behind the designer changes and the effect that those changes imparted lead the foundation of success of this prosthesis and hence needs further elaboration.

The bipolar endoprosthesis consist of polished femoral head prosthesis with a locking internal ultra high molecular weight polyethylene (UHMWPE) bearing that mates with the head of a conventional femoral component.

This design evolved in an effort to palliate certain limitations of the presently used Indian Bipolar. Specific problems encountered over the years with the bipolar system include:-

1. *A very low seating angle makes it mandatory to sacrifice the calcar for proper seating of the prosthesis. This eventually contributes to sinkage of prosthesis and failure.*
2. *Movement of the limb is relatively restricted due to neck impingement at the margin of the cup. This also leads to UHMWPE wear and debris*

formation which contributes to osteolysis, prosthetic loosening, sinkage and stiffness of movement at the inner bearing.

3. *Cementing is not possible with its stem design.*
4. *In this part of the country the Indian bipolar is available only in odd number head sizes. Thus an accurate fit is often not possible and this leads to early chondrolysis. A slightly loose cup in the acetabulum will results in high value of Hertzian contact-stress (Hertz's analysis). On the other hand even a 0.2 mm larger diameter of the steel cup will lead to stresses at the acetabular cartilage in the order of 842.8kpa/ cm^2. These stresses lead to early chondrolysis, acetabular erosions and protrusio. Ultimately this causes prosthesis failure.*
5. *The head size of femoral component is 26mm and a lack of positive eccentricity retards the movement between the metallic head and the UHMWPE contributing to less movement at the inner bearing.*
6. *Conversion of the presently used Indian Bipolar to a total hip system is not possible without removing the whole assembly.*

Due to these short comings in the previous studies done on bipolar found following problems

- Works like Unipolar in two to three years time. *Verberne GHM(1983) J Bone Joint Surg [Br] 72:788-793. Christiansen, Bateman, Giliberty & Monk prosthesis.*
- High Dislocation rates equal to unipolar. *Long JW, Knight W (1980) Bateman UPF prosthesis in fractures of femoral neck. Clin Orhtop 152:198–201*
- Less degree of movement. *Drinker H, Murray WR. J Bone Joint Surg [Am] 1979;61-A:1167-74.*
- Acetabular erosion after 5 years was found to be equivalent to unipolar with previous Bipolar Designs. *Soreide O, Molster A, Raugstad TS (1980) Replacement with the Christiansen endoprosthesis in acute femoral neck fractures: a 5 year follow up study. Acta Orthop Scand 51:137–144.*
- Polyethylene debris shredding due to neck cup impingement. Wear debris from Bipolar femoral neck cup impingement. *J Arthoplasty 1994 Feb 9(1): 89-93*
- Thin layer of polyethylene causes early revision surgery.
- Lack of positive eccentricity. *Krein S.W., Chao E.Y.S. J. orthop. Res 2: 356-368, 1984.*
- Sacrifice of calcar leads to sinkage of prosthesis and failure. Gingras MB, Clarke J, Evarts CM (1980). Clin Orthop 152:147-157.

The BHU Hip device tries to address these problems in a rational ways:

1. **Ellipsoidal outer cup :**The ellipsoidal outer cup provides extremes of the movement and does not dislocate.The patient can sit cross legged and squat due to ellipsoidal shape of it's outer cup.

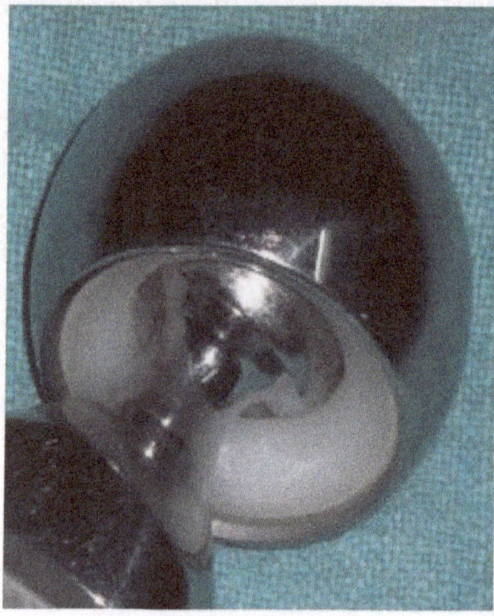

(a)

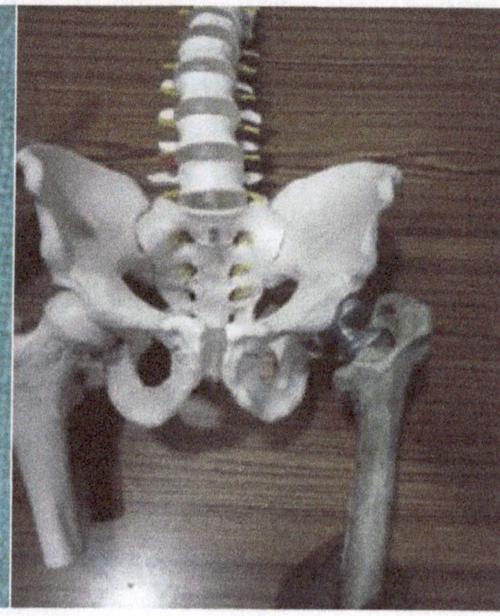

(b)

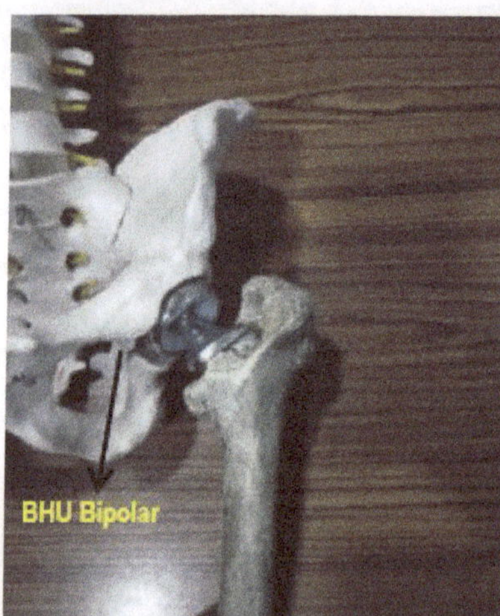

(c)

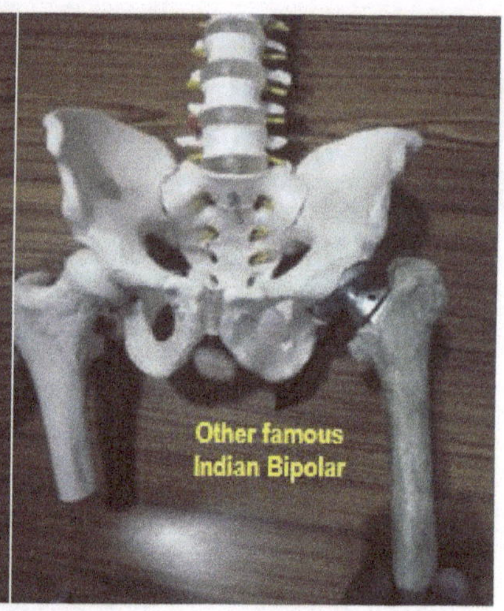

(d)

Note: Figure (a),(b),(c) are in model pictures of BHU Bipolar clearly demonstrating the ellipsoidal cup of prosthesis. Figure (d) is another famous Indian bipolar as difference clearly seen that the head is completely sinked in acetabulum making it prone for dislocation, and chances of neck cup impingement in early range of motions also noticeable

1. The seating angle has been made as anatomical as possible and thus the calcar need not to be sacrificed. Preventing sinking and stress shielding.As continuous sinking of prosthesis in femoral canal has been attributed to early failure of prosthesis.

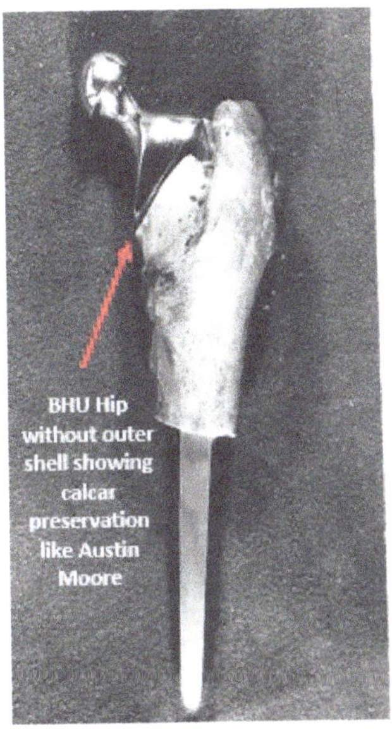
BHU Hip
without outer
shell showing
calcar
preservation
like Austin
Moore

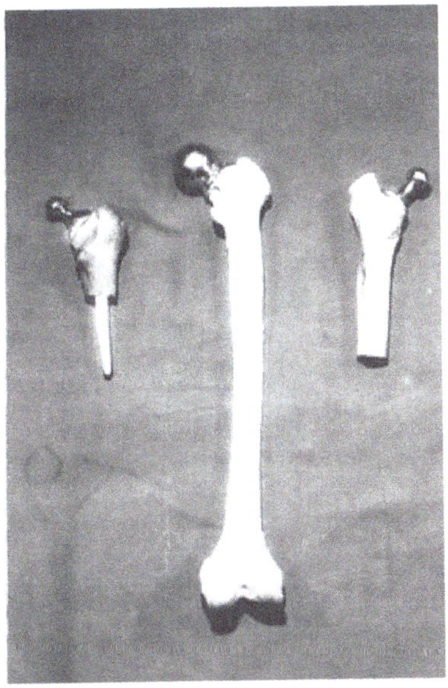

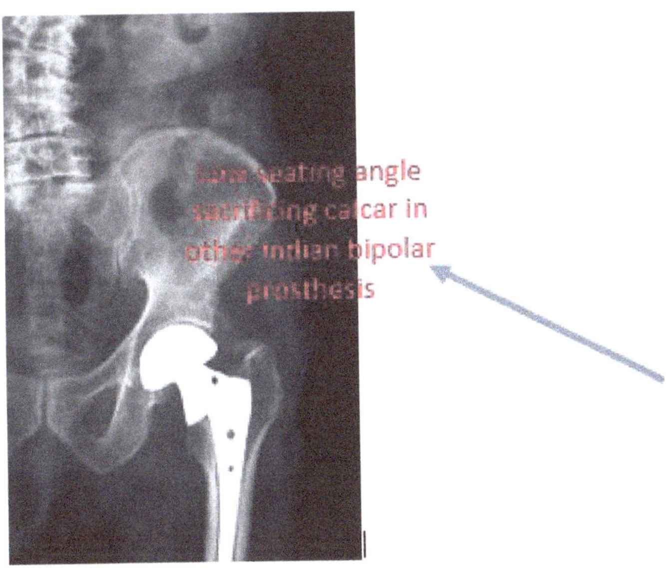

2. The UHMWPE lining has a bevelled margin in a staggering fashion. Thus at the extremes of movement, the neck impinges on the metal cup and not on the UHMWPE lining therefore reducing wear and debris formation, a major cause of failure of most bipolar design.

As seen earlier, various studies have found the debris formation inside the joint as the major cause for bipolar to start acting as unipolar. The shredded debri elicits an inflammatory response leading to fibrosis and cessation at the inner bearing movement.

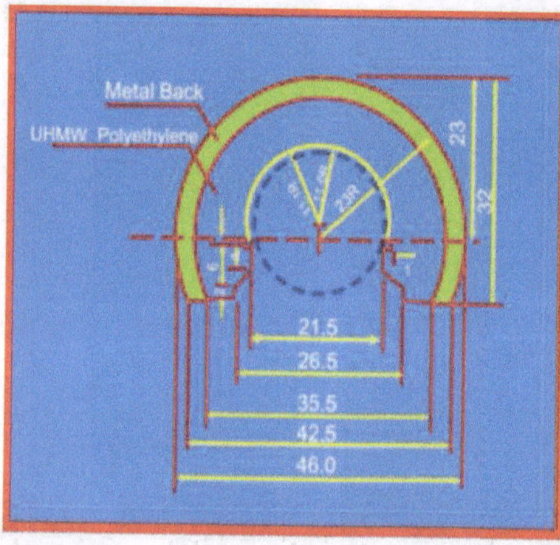

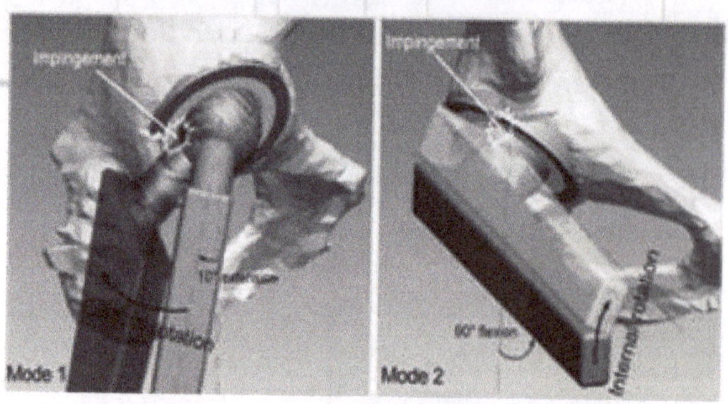

Neck – Cup Impingm ent

3. The neck of the prosthesis has been made trapezoidal like Charnley type neck. This shape of neck as been found to be associated with greater degree of freedom of movement without impingement with cup or polyethylene lining hence reduces the impingement to great extent.

It is evident that outer movement i.e. the movement between acetabulum and cup starts occurring when the neck impinges to either cup or the polyethylene linning in early range of motion, thus cup has been modified in staggering fashion. Since it is the outer movement between the acetabulum and cup that is responsible for acetabular erosion and protrusion, pushing an elderly patient to revison surgery.

4. The inner metallic head has been sized to 22mm unlike 28 or 32 mm in most of other bipolars. The rationale being as seen in chapter of mathematical calculation for given load W, the frictional torque is proportional to the product of coefficient of friction and **radius of hemispherical surface** thus a smaller head is associated with lesser frictional torque.**The smaller diameter head** provides a better positive eccentricity leading to valgus torque instead of varus and increased friction on outer surface compared to inner.

Reducing the head diameter of the inner ball to 22mm provides the benefit of positive eccentricity has . This also provides a greater range of movements between the metallic head and the UHMWPE, thus providing greater percentage of movement at the inner bearing for a longer time and longevity to the system

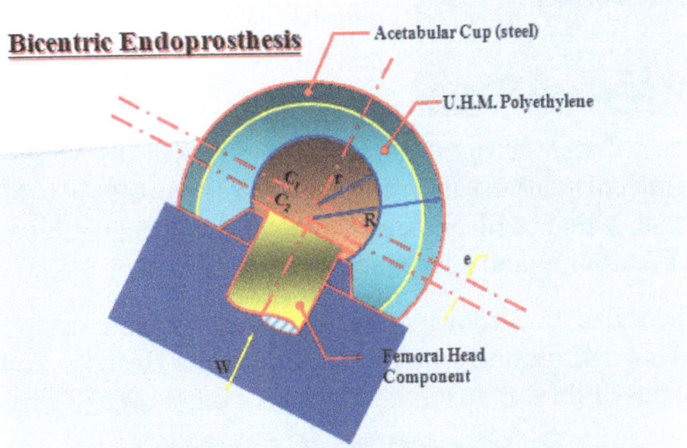

$M_t = (\pi.W/2).\mu.r$ for given load W, the frictional torque is proportional to the product of coefficient of friction and radius of hemispherical surface.

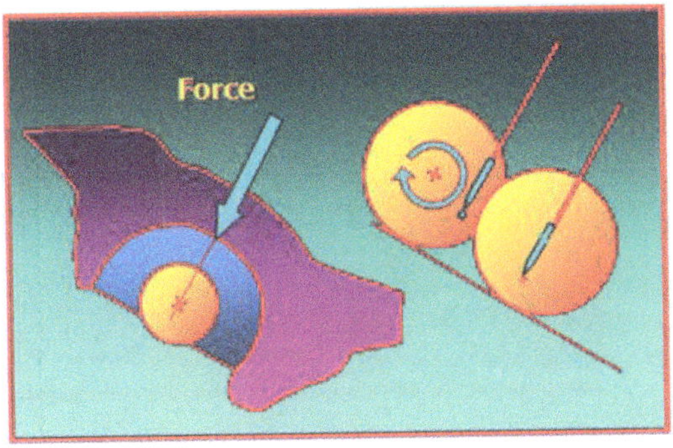

- Wear rate of UHMWPE in a bipolar is 0.21 ± 0.17. *A. Kusba, Y. Kuroki from Showa University Fujigaoka Hospital, Yokohama, JapanJ Bone Joint Surg [Br] 1997;79-B:331-6.Received 2September 1996; Accepted after revision 23 December 1996*

Thus a thicker UHMWPE ensures a longer life of inner lining hence better serviceability of prosthesis.

Due to smaller head of 22mm it has also become possible to accommodate a thicker UHMWPE with greater longevity.

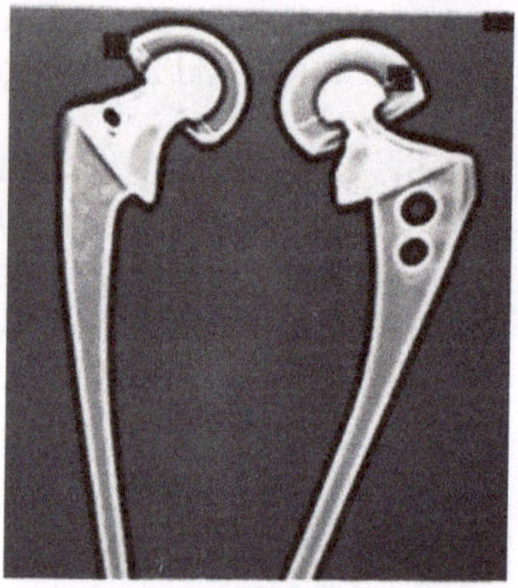

Bicentric bipolar prosthesis (right side) showing increased thickness of UHMWPE due to smaller diameter of the inner head.

Available in 37 to 55 head **sizes in 1 mm increments,** which ensures that the exact required head size as needed on OT table is available on as many occasions as possible and hence prevents use of inappropriate head sizes.

If the steel cup chosen for fitting inside acetabulum is loose or tight, it can be shown (as discussed in chapter of mathematical calculation) that this will result to a high value of Hertzian contact stress, which will be detrimental to the cartilage layer at the inside surface of acetabulumand subsequently early failure of the prosthesis.

Thus the had size in 1 mm increment allows,accurate acetabular fit and a uniform stress distribution which also avoids the Hertzian contact stress, so lessens the possibility of *cartilage degeneration, pain and protrusio.*

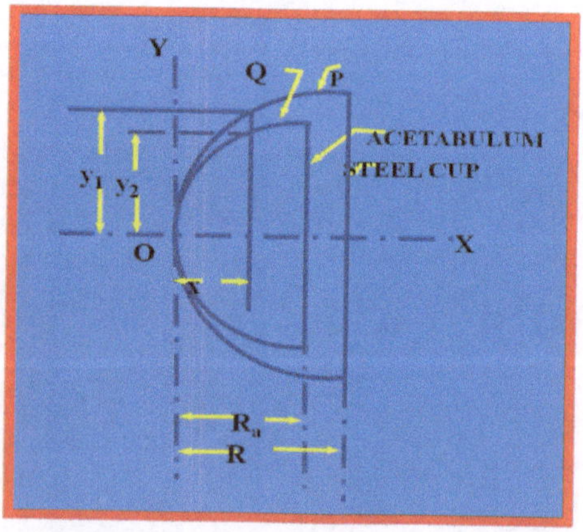

Effect of stress on acetabulum even with 1mm discrepancy of head size is substantial.

Based on the calculation for200 pounds (890 N) men various stress in acetabulum

-Snug fit cup 1.345 Mpa (13.71 Kg/cm^2)

-For Loose cup 17.72 MPa (180.63Kg/cm^2)

-For Tight cup 51.2 Mpa (521.9 Kg/cm^2)

If the steel cup chosen for fitting inside acetabulum is loose, it can be shown that this will result to a high value of Hertzian contact stress, which will be detrimental to the cartilage layer at the inside surface of acetabulum. Such a loose fit of steel cup is shown in Fig.

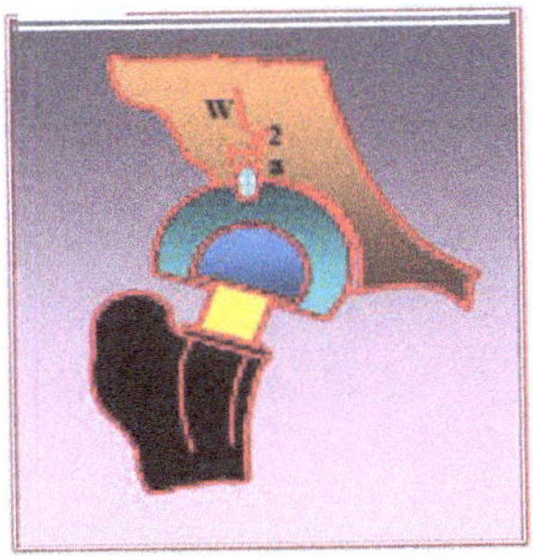

$$a = \sqrt[3]{(3W/4).[\{(1-v_s^2)/E_s\} + \{(1-v_b^2)/E_b\}] / [(1/R)-(1/R_a)]}$$

Where 2R = diameter of steel cup. $2R_a$ = diameter of inside surface of acetabulum, W = load transmitted through the system, v_s & E_s = poisson's ratio and the elasticity modulus of steel, . V_b, E_b = poisson's ratio and the elasticty modulus of bone, a = radius of circular contact area

Hertz 's analysis

Articulating and disarticulating jigs have been designed and trialled to make the system more versatile. Conversion of the bipolar hemiarthroplasty to total hip arthroplasty is cost effective and less time consuming, as the femoral component does not require to be replaced.

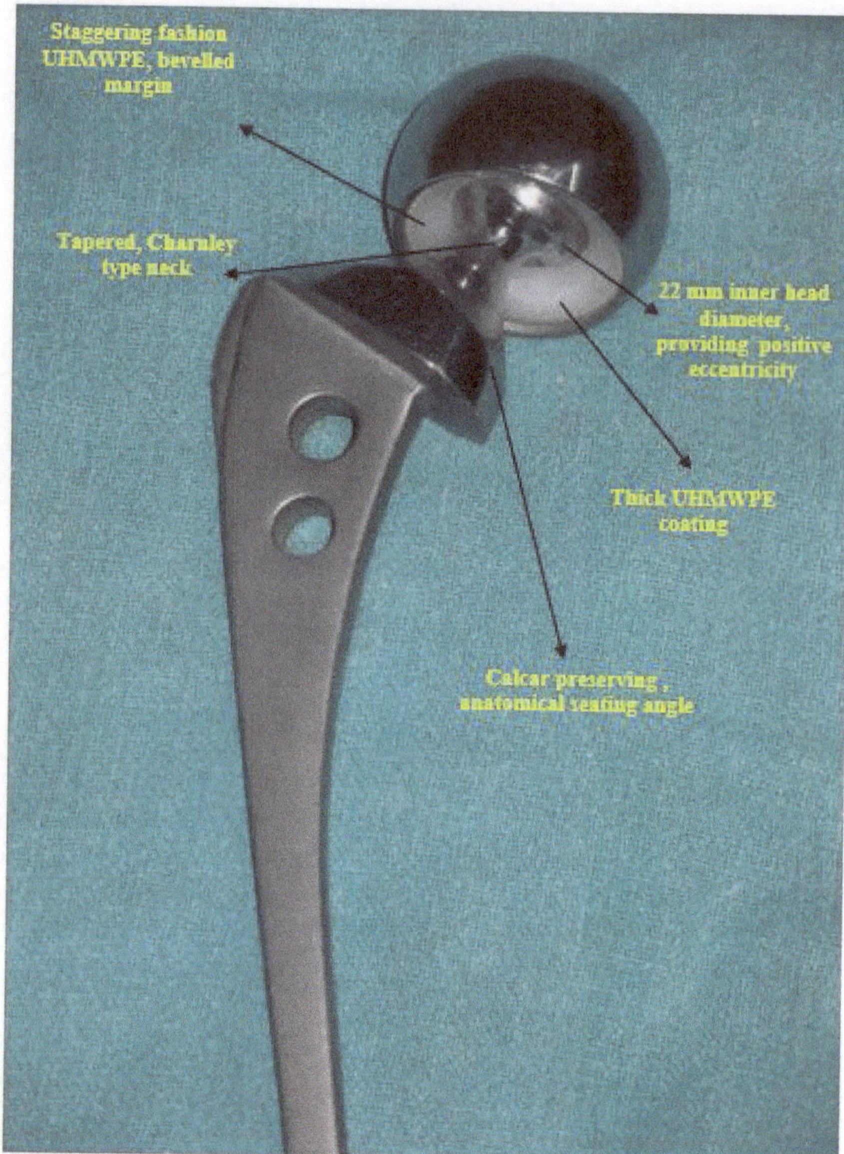
Staggering fashion UHMWPE, bevelled margin
Tapered, Charnley type neck
22 mm inner head diameter, providing positive eccentricity
Thick UHMWPE coating
Calcar preserving , anatomical seating angle

REFERENCES

1. Kobayashi S; Takaoka K; Tsukada A; Ueno M: Polyethylene wear from femoral bipolar neck-cup impingement as a cause of femoral prosthetic loosening. 21 : Arch Orthop Trauma Surg 1998;117(6-7) : 390-1.

2. Kiekens G; Somville J; Taminiau A: Clinical relevance of acetabular erosion in young patients with a bipolar hip prosthesis. 12: Acta Orthop Belg 2000 Dec;66(5) : 455-60

3. Kusaba A; Kuroki Y: Wear of bipolar hip prostheses. J Arthroplasty, 13:668-73, 1998 Sep.

4. Messieh M; Mattingly DA; Turner RH; Scott R; Fox J; Slater J: Wear debris from bipolar femoral neck-cup impingement. A case of femoral stem loosening. 35: J Arthroplasty 1994 Feb; 9(1):89-93.

5. Mollers M; Stedtfeld HW; Paechtner S, Wald A: Hemi-arthroplasty of the hip joint: concentric or positive eccentric (self-centering) dual head prosthesis: a retrospective comparison. 38:Unfallchirurg 1992 M

6. Tsukamoto Y; Mabuchi K; Futami T; Kubotera D: Motion of the bipolar hip prosthesis components. Friction studied in cadavers. Acta Orthop Scand, 63:648-52, 1992 Decay;95(5):224-9.

7. Bartz R L, Noble P C, Kadakia N R, Tullos H S. The effect of femoral component head size on posterior dislocation of the artifi cial hip joint. J Bone Joint Surg (Am) 2000; 82 (9): 1300-7

8. Verberne GHM(1983) J Bone Joint Surg [Br] 72:788-793. Christiansen, Bateman, Giliberty & Monk prosthesis.

9. Soreide O, Molster A, Raugstad TS (1980) Replacement with the Christiansen endoprosthesis in acute femoral neck fractures: a 5 year follow up study. Acta Orthop Scand 51:137–144.

10. Krein S.W., Chao E.Y.S. J. orthop. Res 2: 356-368, 1984.

11. A. Kusba, Y. Kuroki from Showa University Fujigaoka Hospital, Yokohama, JapanJ Bone Joint Surg [Br] 1997;79-B:331-6.

12. Gingras MB, Clarke J, Evarts CM (1980). Clin Orthop 152:147-157.

THE MATHMATICAL ANALYSIS

Bicentric Endoprosthesis, advantage of positive eccentricity

A normal occasionally high body weight results into the transmission of force W through the femoral neck to the head component. Any movement of lower limb under this will give rise to frictional force between the metal and the internal spherical surface of ultra high molecular weight, polyethylene, with a frictional torque about the center $C_1$of head component. It is the same force 'W' that transmits to the acetabular cup and there develops a frictional force between the outer metallic cup and the inner surface of the acetabulum.

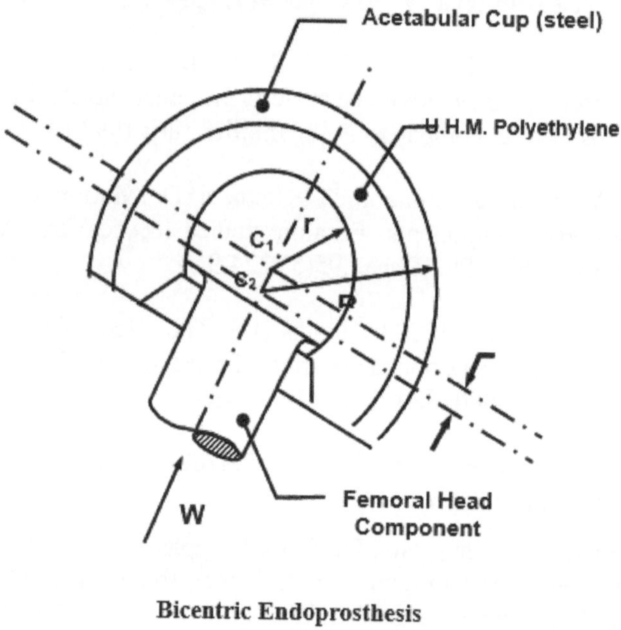

Bicentric Endoprosthesis

A frictional torque is produced when the loaded hip moves through an arc of motion. It is the product of the friction force times the length of the lever arm that is, the distance given point on surface or the head moves during a given arc of motion.

Relation between the Applied Force and Pressure

A relation between the applied force W and the pressure over the assumed hemispherical surface is obtained with reference to Fig., which is explained below:

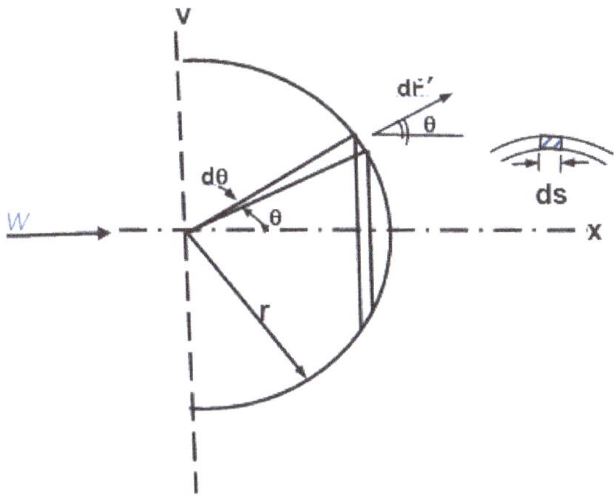

Elementary area, $dA' = r.d\theta.\ ds$

Elementary force $dF' = p.dA' = p.r.d\theta.\ ds,$

Where p = pressure (force per unit area) which is assumed to be uniformly distributed over the entire hemispherical surface.

Axial component $\quad dF = dF'.Cos\theta = p.r.Cos\theta.d\theta.ds$

Hence, the axial force due to the pressure on the elementary ring is written as,

$$dF_a = (p.r.Cos\theta.d\theta)(2\pi r.Sin\theta)$$

or, $$dF_a = p.2\pi r^2.Sin\theta.Cos\theta.d\theta$$

Total axial force, $$F_a = \int df_a = p.2\pi r^2 . \int_0^{\pi/2} Sin\theta.Cos\theta.d\theta$$

or, $\mathbf{F_a = W = p.\pi.r^2}$

Hence, the pressure $\mathbf{p = W/\pi r^2}$ ....

Frictional Torque

Frictional torque develops due to frictional force at the hemispherical surfaces.

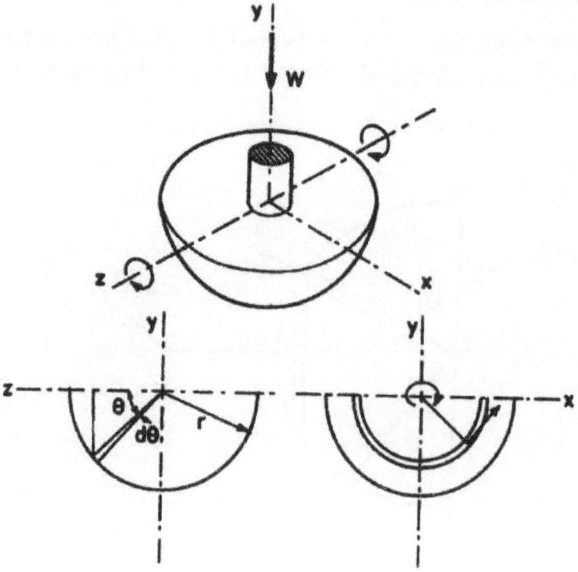

Elementary area = (r.dθ) (π.r.Sinθ) = π.r². Sinθ.dθ

Elementary frictional torque, $dM_t = \mu.p.(\pi r^2.\text{Sin}\theta.d\theta)\,(r.\text{Sin}\theta)$

Total frictional torque, $M_t = 2\mu.p.\pi r^3 \int_0^{\pi/2} \text{Sin}^2\theta.d\theta$

or, $M_t = \mu.p.(\pi^2/2)r^3$

Using $p = W/\pi r^2$, $M_t = (\pi.W/2).\mu.r$

It is found that for any given load 'W', the frictional torque is proportional to the product of coefficient of friction and radius of hemispherical surface.

Comparison of rotational movements

Since the same load acts axially through the neck of the femoral component, the pressure between the head component and the UHMW polyethylene cavity as seen in the figure below :

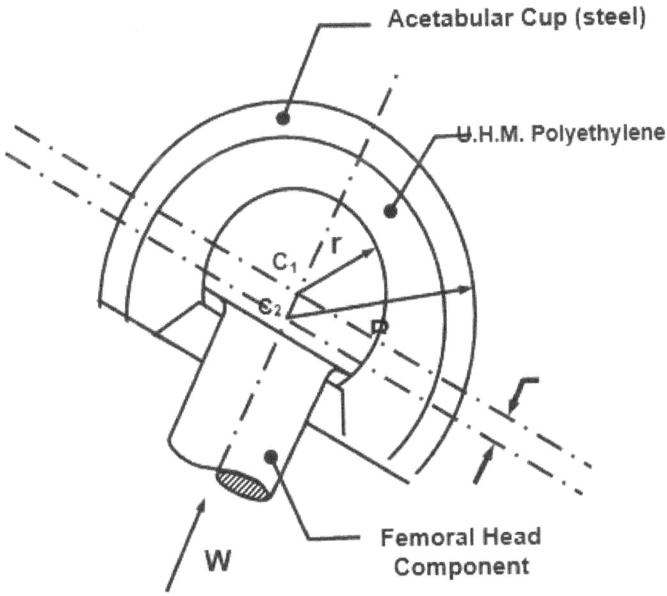

is obtained as –

$$p_1 = W/\pi.r^2$$

Where r = radius of the spherical head element

Similarly, the pressure between the cup and the acetabulum is

$$p_2 = W/\pi.R^2$$

Where R = radius of spherical surfaces of the metallic cup and the acetabulum assuming that the cup is snugly fitting in acetabulum. It may be observed that $r<R$, so that $p_2<p_1$.

Further, the tendency of rotation of the head of the femoral element and that of the cup can be explained with the help of frictional torque associated with each of these two. The rotation of head element within the U.H.M.W. polyethylene cavity will occur at a limiting frictional torque.

$$M_{t1} = (\pi.W/2).\mu_h.r,$$

Where μ_h = coefficient of friction between the metallic head of femoral element and U.H.M.W. polyethylene, and r = radius of head element. If the femoral head component would have been integral with the cup, the limiting value of frictional torque would have been

$$M_{t2} = (\pi.W/2).\mu_c.R,$$

Where μ_c = coefficient of friction between the cup and acetabulum.

The desired effect, i.e. the head of femoral component rotates before the cup's rotation in the acetabulum, is achieved due to the positive eccentricity, e = R-r, and the favourable condition for this will be

$$Mt1 < Mt2$$

$$\text{or,} \quad \mu_h . r < \mu_c . R$$

$$\text{or,} \quad \mu_c > \mu_h \, (r/R) \quad \ldots\ldots\ldots\ldots (3)$$

In order to prevent wear of the cartilage layer of acetabulum, there should be a minimum movement of metallic cup in the acetabulum. As may be observed from relation above, a condition favouring it depends on μ_h and the ratio (r/R). The coefficient of friction μ_h between the metallic head of femoral prosthesis and the U.H.M.W. polyethylene is found to be close to 0.02. The diameter (2.r) of femoral prosthesis head available are 22, 26 and 32mm, and the diameter (2.R) of metallic cup ranges from 41mm to 55mm. Hence, the selection of both of these matching elements should be such that the ratio (r/R) can be maintained at a small value. It has been reported that synovial fluid is responsible for a low coefficient of friction (0.008 to 0.02) for a normal joint. However, in the absence of synovial fluid, the coefficient of friction between the metallic cup and the acetabulum is likely to be higher. If μ_C is close to but higher than the product μ_h (r/R), there is a greater possibility of rotation of femoral head component within the metallic cup. This is the advantage derived from positive eccentricity in bicentric endoprosthesis.

Stresses in Acetabulum due to Interference Fit of Metallic Cup

If the metallic cup is a little larger in size (diameter) than the internal spherical cavity of the acetabulum, the cup fits into the acetabulum under external load and this becomes a force-fit joint. As a result, the cup either does not rotate in the acetabulum or it may rotate with erosion of cartilage layer. The stress in the bone in close vicinity of the acetabulum is determined as explained below:

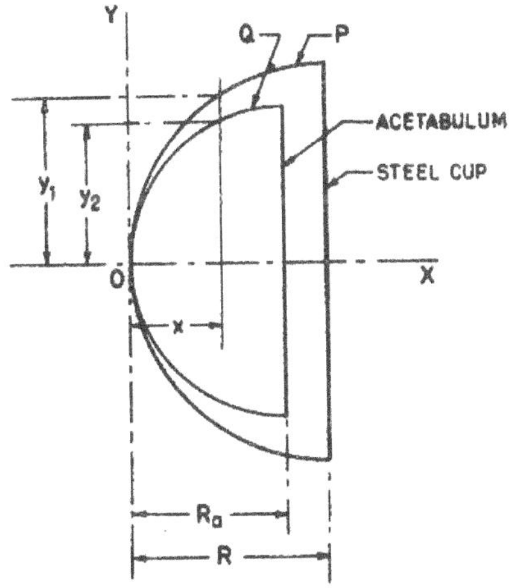

Fig. 12

In Fig 20, a comparison of the size of cup (P) and the acetabulum (Q) is shown schematically in an exaggerated view in which R denotes the radius of metallic cup and 'Ra' denotes the radius of the acetabular cavity. An arbitrary length along the axis of acetabulum is denoted by X. Considering the coordinate system shown in Fig., equations of curves P and Q are

$$Y=\sqrt{R^2-(x-R)^2}, \text{ for P}$$

And $$Y=\sqrt{Ra^2-(x-Ra)^2}, \text{ for Q}$$

Thus, we have $$y_1=x.\sqrt{(2R/x)-1}$$

and as the cup sits in the acetabulum under pressure, it can be assumed that the metallic cup is sufficiently rigid relative to the bone, so that the curve Q in Fig. Assumes the shape of curve P. Hence the circumferencial strain in the bone surrounding the acetabulum becomes

$$\varepsilon=(2\pi y_1-2\pi y_2)/2\pi y_2=(y_1/y_2)-1$$

or, $$\varepsilon=\sqrt{(2R-x)/(2Ra-x)}-1$$

If the acetabulum cavity is assumed to be hemispherical, we have

$$\varepsilon=\sqrt{(2R/Ra)-1}-1$$

Therefore, the circumferential stress = $E.\varepsilon$

$$=E.(\sqrt{(2R/Ra)-1}-1$$

There is, however, some additional circumferential stress due to pressure on the internal surface, which is written as

$$\sigma = p/2 = W/(2.\pi.Ra^2)$$

Hence, the total circumferential stress becomes

$$\sigma = E.(\sqrt{(2R/Ra)-1}-1)+(W/2\pi.Ra^2)$$

Where, E = elasticity modulus of bone.

Application

Reaction force of hip joint

Weight of man (sample) = 200 Ib = 890N

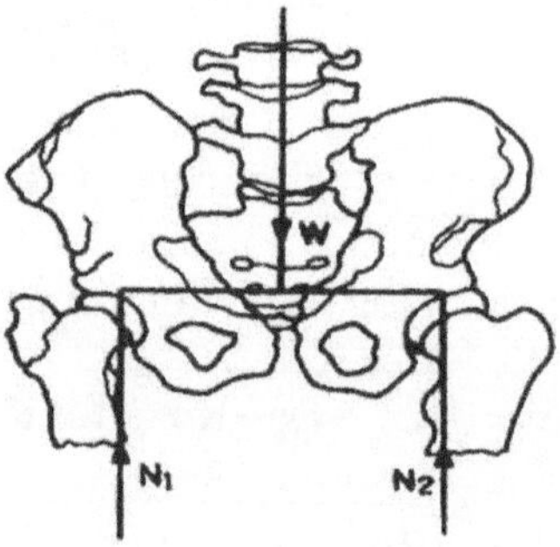

In bilateral stance, the superincumbent weight W passes an equal distance of 6 inches (150mm) between the two hip joints. One lower limb weighs 15.6 per cent of the total body weight. Both lower limbs will be 31.2 per cent of body weight.

$$\therefore \text{Actual load, } W = 890(1-0.312)$$

For, $N_1 = N_2$, and $N_1+N_2 = W$,

$N_1 = N_2 = W/2 = 306.16N$

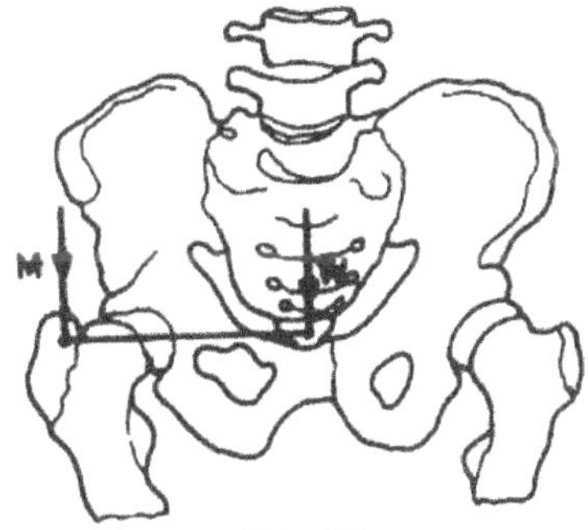

Fig 14

For unilateral stance (see fig.), however, Inman (1947) has estimated the forces and their respective lever arm such that the static compression force on the head of the femur is 2.4 to 2.6 times the body weight.

Therefore, assuming unilateral stance, the force transmitted through the hip joint,

$$W = 2.6\ (1- 0.156).\ 890;N$$

$$= 1953\ N$$

Next, considering a bipolar endoprosthesis system of specification 6924-2-243, having diameter of the steel cup as 43mm and diameter of the femoral head component as 22mm, the pressure at the inside surface of the acetabulum is found to be

$$p = W/\pi.r^2 = 1953/\pi.(21.5 \times 10^{-3})^2 = 1.345\text{Mpa}\ (13.71\text{Kg/cm}^2)$$

Similarly, the maximum frictional torque at the head of femoral component within the steel cup is

$$Mt = (\pi.W/2).\mu h.r = (\pi.1953/2) \times 0.02 \times 11 \times 10^{-3} = 0.675\text{N.m}$$

The value of frictional torque obtained above is much smaller than the moment due to weight W, given by

$$\text{Moment} = W.I. = 1953 \times 150 \times 10^{-3}\ \text{N.m.} = 293\text{N.m}$$

Circumferential Stress at Acetabulum due to Interference Fit of Steel Cup

If the diameter of the acetabular cavity is 42.8mm as compared with 43mm steel cup,

$$R = 21.5\text{mm},\ Ra = 21.4\text{mm},\ E = 17.6 \times 10^9\text{N/m}^2$$

$$\therefore \text{Stress}, \sigma = E.(\sqrt{(2R/Ra)-1}-1) + (W/2\pi Ra^2)$$

$$=17.6\text{x}10^9(\sqrt{(2\text{x}21.5/21.4)-1}-1)$$

$$=+1953/(2\pi(21.4\text{x}10^{-3})^2$$

$$=82.68\text{Mpa}\ (842.8\ \text{Kg/cm}^2)$$

The bone at the acetabulum will be constantly subjected to a stress of above value which is undesirable. A very high stress in bone leads to chondrolysis.

Comparison of stress in acetabulum cartilage in unilateral stance of a patient weighing 200lbs.

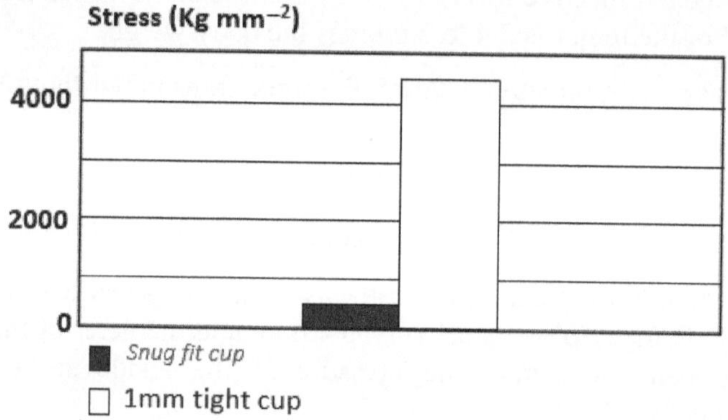

Effect of Loose Steel Cup in Acetabulum

If the steel cup chosen for fitting inside acetabulum is loose, it can be shown that this will result to a high value of Hertzian contact stress, which will be detrimental to the cartilage layer of the acetabulum. Such a loose fit of steel cup is shown in Fig

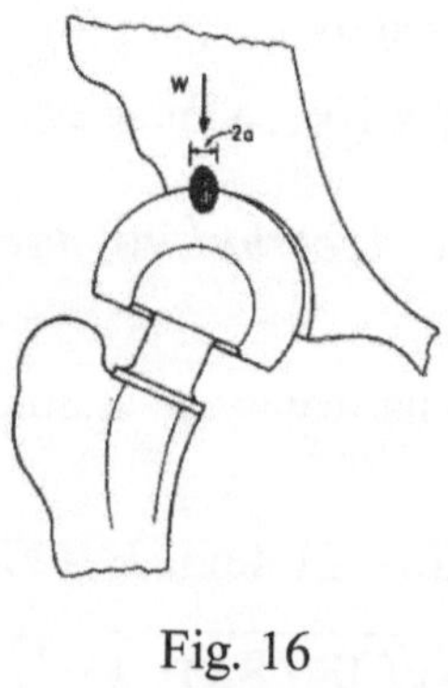

Fig. 16

Comparison of Hertzian contact stress in for a 1mm loose cup in unilateral stance

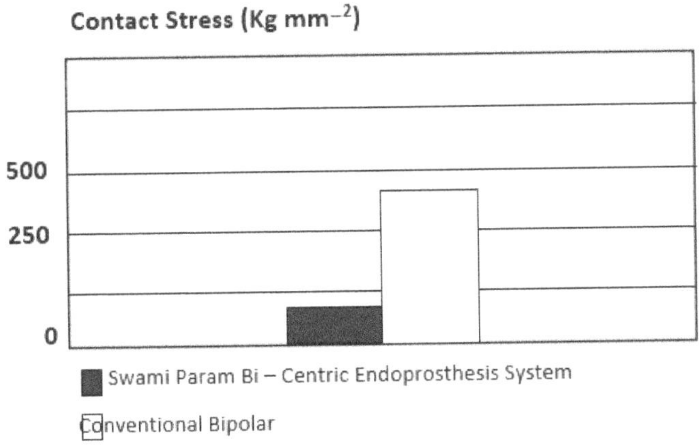

To calculate the Hertz contact stress the following notations are assumed:

2R = diameter of steel cup

2Ra = diameter of inside surface of acetabulum

W = load transmitted through the system

ν_S, E_S = Poisson's ratio and the elasticity modulus of steel

ν_S, E_b = Poisson's ratio and the elasticity modulus of bone

a = radius of circular contact area

As the steel cup under the effect of load presses against the inside surface of acetabulum, the radius of the circular contact area is obtained according to Hertz's analysis[3] as

$$A=\sqrt[3]{(3W/4).[\{1-\nu_s^2)/E_s\}+\{(1-\nu_b^2)/E_b\}]/[(1/R)-(1/Ra)]}$$

Hence, the maximum pressure at the contact area is written as

$$p_{max} = 3W/2\pi a^2$$

Application

For a load of 1953 N as the extreme load condition in unilateral stance, the other required data are as follows:

$\nu_S = 0.3$, $E_S = 206$Gpa, $\nu_b = 0.3$, $E_b = 17.6$Gpa,

R = 21.5mm, Ra = 21.6mm (a loose cup)

Hence, the radius of circular contact area

$$\sqrt{\frac{\frac{(3x1953)}{4} x[\{\frac{1-0.3)^2}{206}\}+\{\frac{(1-0.3)^2}{17.6}\}]}{\frac{1}{21.5}-(1-21.6)}}$$

Or, $a = 7.2543 \text{ x } 10^{-3}\text{m}$

∴ Maximum pressure $= 3 \text{ x } 1953 \text{ x } 10^6/2\pi\ (7.2543)2;\text{N/m}^2$

$= 17.72\text{Mpa } (180.63\text{Kg/cm}^2)$

Thus, the maximum pressure is much higher than a pressure of 1.345Mpa for the cases of a snug fit cup.

Also, with 2R = 43mm and 2Ra = 44mm, we have,

$a = 4.2684 \text{ x } 10^{-3}\text{m}$, and $p_{max} = 51.2\text{Mpa } (521.9 \text{ Kg/cm}^2)$

Conclusion

1. **A slight loose cup is less damaging to the acetabular cartilage than a tight cup. However, a loose cup will not provide the benefit of positive eccentricity and the desired rotation between the head of femoral component and the outer cup.**

2. **A tight cup results into a greater movement between 22mm diameter. Head of femoral component and the U.H.M.W. polyethylene lining of cup but the overall stress on the acetabular cartilage will be highly damaging in the long run.**

3. **A 22mm diameter head of femoral component is preferable to a 26mm diameter head from the standpoint of positive eccentricity, which is missing in the present bipolar system available in this country.**

NON-CEMENTED VARIETY OF STEM

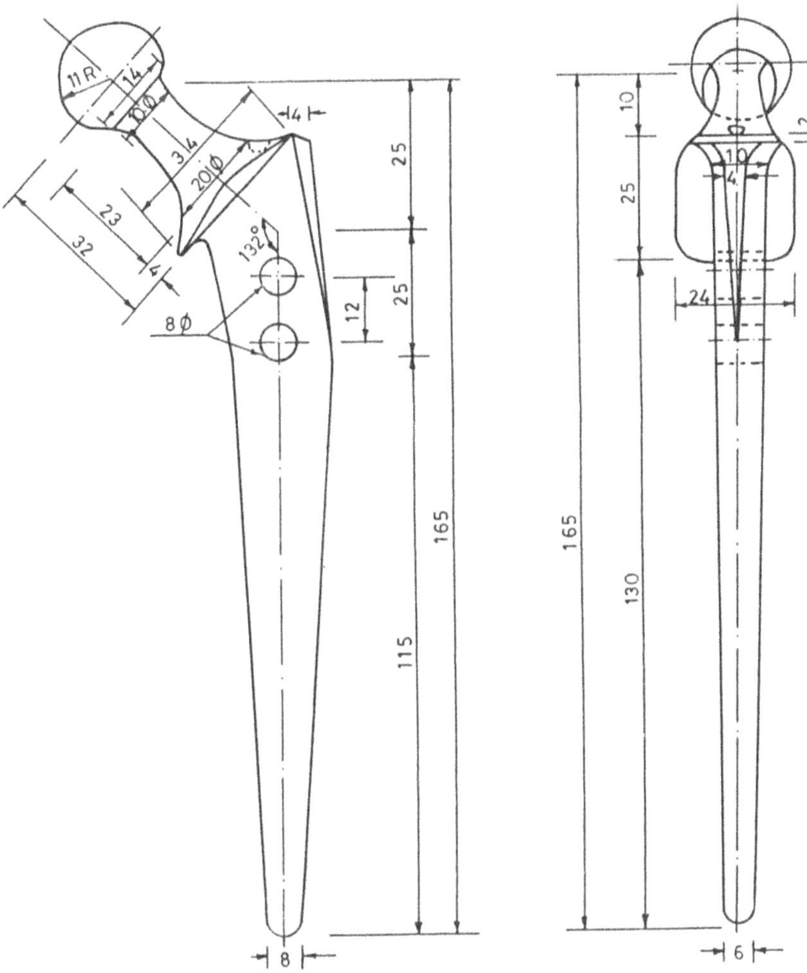

Ultra - High Molecular Weight Polyethylene Cup With Supper Finish Metal Back

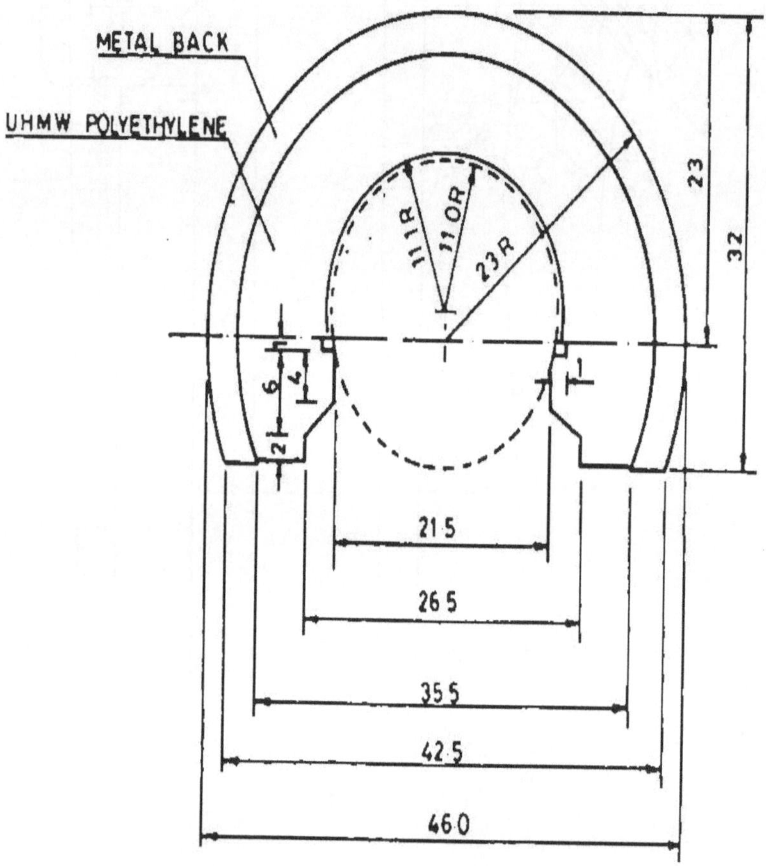

RESULTS

From the very beginning of its existence bipolar prosthesis was the subject of debate, many researches and trials were done to test the idea behind the generation of prosthesis and different researchers gave different result with most researches opine that the bipolar process is no better than unipolar hemiarthroplasty**. Verberne** et all in early 1986 in his study concluded that the bipolar prosthesis(vericoff prosthesis used by him) starts acting as unipolar in span of three months hence no more better than unipolar, similarly**Drinker and Murray** using Universal proximal femoral prosthesis in their study of hemi replacement in fracture neck of femur and in osteonecrosis in 1979 published that they noted far less inner bearing motion then allowed by prosthesis itself and in addition they also found that there was a gradual decrease in inner bearing movement. They in their conclusion said that bipolar prosthesis should be reserved for the patients younger than 70 year with head problem but no marked acetabular involvement.In same year however **Lestrange** in his four year review of batsman prosthesis found out that this prosthesis provides definitive advantage over unipolar prosthesis.**Hebeck et al** in their 4 year RCT between bipolar hemiarthroplasty and total hip arthroplasty for displaced neck femur fracture reported that total hip arthroplasty was associated with better hip function as compared with bipolar. In 2012 **Lihong Fan** compared bipolar hemiarthroplasty with total hip replacement for unstable intertrochanteric fractures in elderly osteoporotic patients and reported that bipolar is better recommended then total hip arthroplasty in terms of cost, duration of surgery and blood loss, as the hip function was not significantly different for the two.

In 2019 New England Journal of Medicine publish that among independently ambulating patients with displaced fracture neck of femur incidence of secondary procedure does not differ between total hip arthroplasty and bipolar arthroplasty and there was no significant advantage of total hip arthroplasty in terms of function for quality of life.

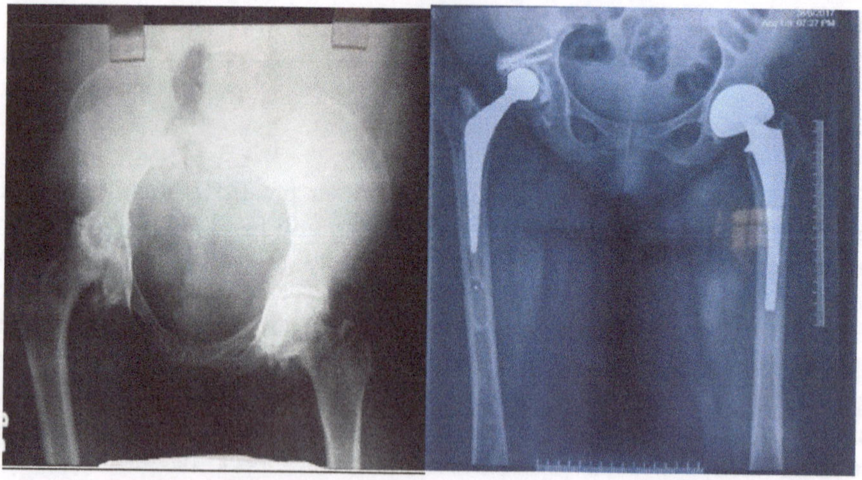

A case of bilateral AVN hip in 65 year female treated with THR (**Tx cost-1,50000 ,OT duration-2 hrs, 5% dislocation rate**) on right side and BHU bipolar on left side (**25,000, OT duration 45 mins, No incidence of dislocation**)

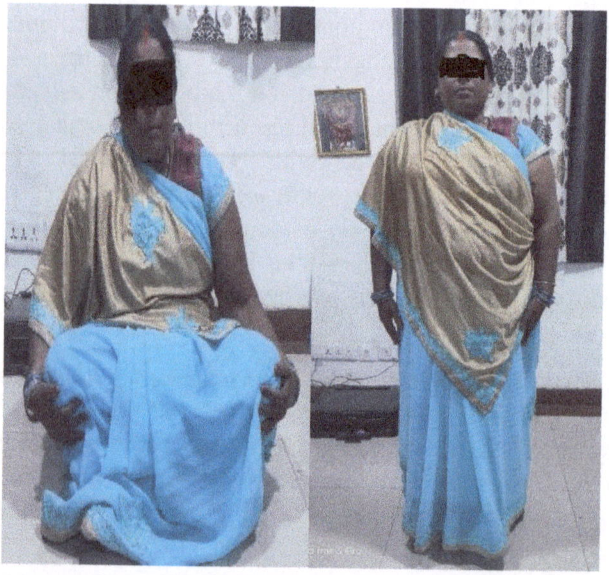

Patient is subjectively more comfortable on left hip i.e. side where Bipolar prosthesis was put.

Above mentioned case clearly demonstrates that a well designed Bipolar prosthesis can very well narrow down the indications for use of a Total Hip Replacement.

At our institute from 2007 to 2009 we performed total of 210 hemiarthroplasty using the uncemented BHU bipolar device, out of which 158 was performed for fresh fracture neck of femur and 52 were done for arthritic hip due to various causes with not severe acetabular involvement and we assessed the performance of this device on following mentioned parameters

1. **Harris hip score**
2. **Radiological assessment of Inner bearing movement**
3. **Incidence of clinical and radiological complications**

Harris hip score was calculated at 1st year post op, followed by 5 years and 10 years post op follow up and there was a gradual decrease in the overall hip scoring as shown in the table below

	Arthritic hip	**Neck femur fracture**
1 yr post op	86.79 + 3.51	87.5+ 4.19
5 yr post op	82.81 + 7.74	85.64 + 3.49
10 yr post op	79. 42 + 5.86	80.37 + 2.98

Hemiarthroplasty done for fresh neck femur fracture demonstrated slightly better Harris hip score then done for arthritic hip however the difference is insignificant (p> .001). Similarly the decrease in Harris hip score from period of 1 to 5 yrs post-op and from 5 to 10 yrs post op was also insignificant however the decrease from 1st to 10 yrs post-op was significant.

Patient Personal opinion

Out of all the patients **78%** rated the surgery as very good, while 12% patients opined that the procedure is good enough, 8 % patients said that they are satisfied with the surgery, however 2 % of total patient were not satisfied by the procedure. Most of these unsatisfied patients were those who were having problems from longer duration and somehow had adjusted with their symptoms hence surgery does not mad much of change in their lifestyle.

Contractures- There was no significant difference in incidence and extent of contracture between operated and contralateral non operated hip. Thus establishing a successful serviceability of prosthesis.

Infection and other morbity – There were 6 cases of infection. 4 of them were superficial infection with serous or serosanguinous discharge for which culture and sensitivity was done and treated subsequently with regular dressing and antibiotics.

While two patients had deep infection and the infection presented during 2nd post op week as wound dehiscence, extending up to periprosthetic space which required arthrotomy, lavage and closure over a drain which was removed 3 days following surgery. These patients had a significant decrease in range of motion and functional outcome as compared to others.

Setting of prosthesis/Prosthesis subsidence referred to a reduction of 5 mm of the distance between the apex of the lesser trochanter and medial apex of femoral stem. Only 7 of total patients showed up recordable setting of prosthesis. Range of motion and functional outcome however was not significantly different from those not having setting of prosthesis.

None of the patient showed any radiological or clinical evidence of loosening of prosthesis as suggested by presence of ≤1 mm periprosthetic radiolucent lines that were continuous and parallel to the prosthesis while there was no progressive displacement and no presence of new varus and valgus, or appearance of separation of porous surface or prosthetic fracture.

There was no incidence of any prosthetic dislocation and only two patients required revision surgery because of the deep seated infection as mentioned earlier.

None of the patient had intolerable or intractable pain at any period of follow up that suggested there was no progressive arthritis of acetabulum.

Thirty one patients of total used some kind of support while walking.

Acetabular protrusion – There was no significant increase in acetabular protrusion during the follow up with a mean of 6 mm (ranging from 3- 15 mm). However the pain score for the patient was not significantly different compared with pain score for patients w/o protrusion, similarly the range of motion was also not significantly different in patient with acetabular protrusion compared to patient without protrusion.

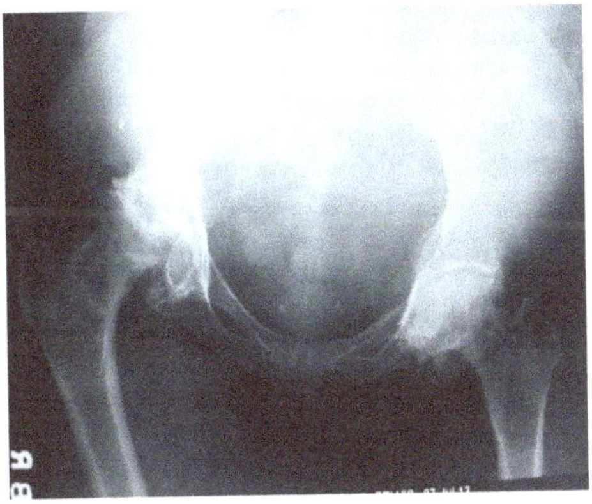

36 yr old female patient came to us with this challenging X ray. Obvious choice, go ahead with THR, however we performed a staged hemi replacement .

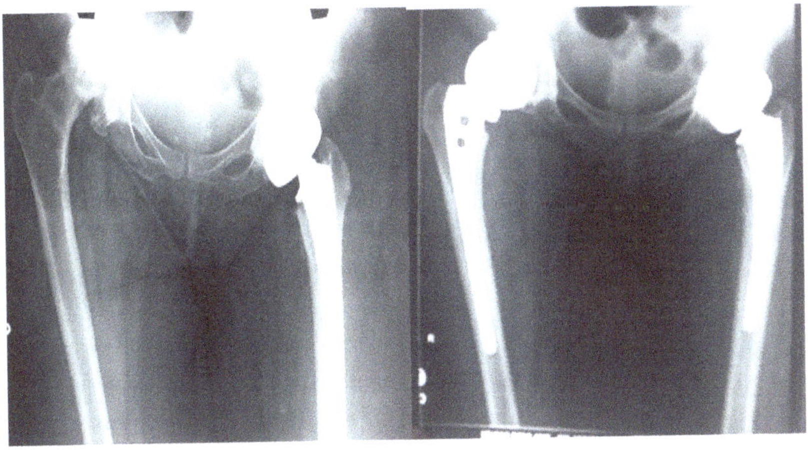

Left Hip was operated first with BHU Bipolar prosthesis	Right hip was operated 1 month after the left one. Acetabulum was reamed to have a socket at

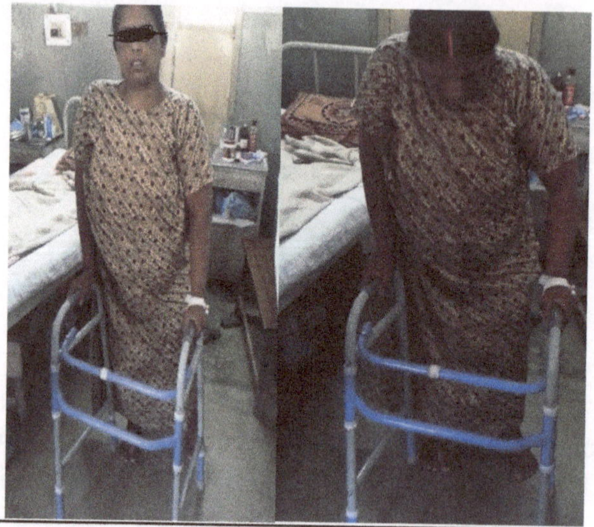

Same 36 yr old female patient with bilateral hip involvement and BHU prosthesis in situ.

Results like these have encouraged us to extend the indication beyond the boundaries earlier set by previous bipolar designs and provided a cost effective yet very reliable option for such patients.

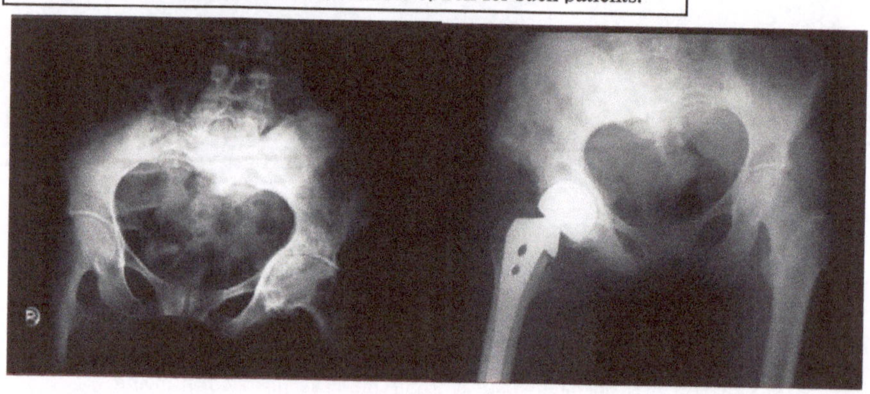

55 years female case of advanced Tubercular arthritis with stiff & painful hip. 14 yrs post op: no acetabular protrusion , clinically no restriction of ROM (***worth mentioning that all studies in past found that almost all bipolar start acting as unipolar with in 1 yr leading to acetabular erosion and protrusion***)

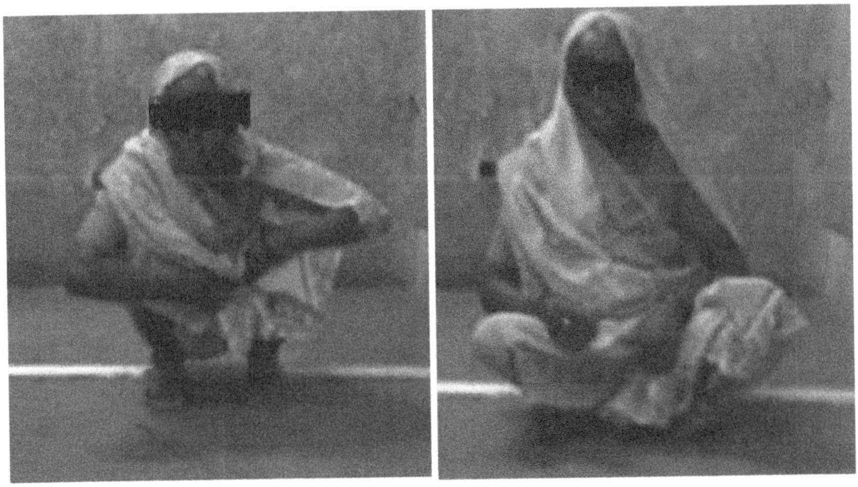

Inner bearing movement

Idea of bipolar prosthesis has been to shift the movement from metal to bone interface to metal on polyethylene interface to tackle the problem of acetabular erosion associated with unipolar prosthesis, but right from beginning of its existence it was put to scrutiny. As mentioned earlier in this chapter that there have been studies in past that contradicted the idea of bipolarity in prosthesis. While there are studies that tell that it is a successful device with good long term outcome and then there are studics that put it equivalent to total hip replacements.

Radiological evaluation assessing contribution of each surface in total movement was done by using method as acquired by Bochner RM et al.Antero–posterior x–rays of both hips were taken with the patient first in neutral and then in maximum abduction. A line drawn tangential to the most inferior aspects of the ischia was used as a reference line. Angle A^1- was defined by the intersection of reference line with line drawn along the inferior margin of the acetabular component in neutral position. Angle B^1 was formed by the intersection of the ischial reference line with a line drawn along the center of the long axis of the femoral stem in neutral position. The exercise was repeated on the x-ray in fully abducted position and angles A^2 and B^2 were found.

The difference between angle B^2 and B^1 i.e. B^3 represented the total abduction taking place at the operated hip. Change between A^2 and A^1 i.e. A^3 represented the amount of motion taking place between the metal and the acetabulum. The difference between B^3- A^3 represented the amount of abduction taking place at the inner bearing.

Thus the total amount of abduction and its outer and inner components were calculated and tabulated for each patient at each follow up.

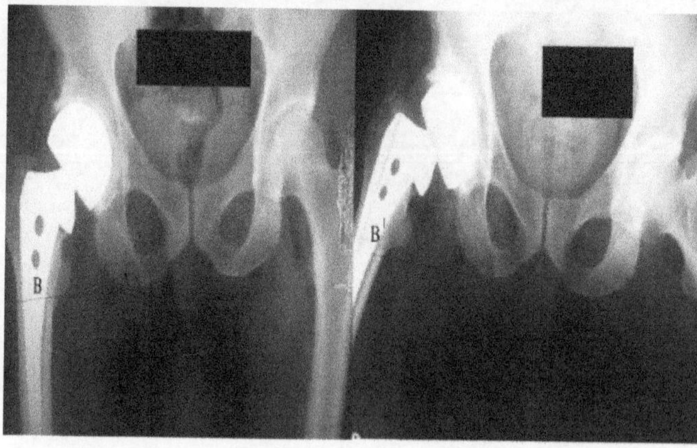

Angle B^3= (B^2-B^1) = Amount of abduction **(Total)**

Angle A^3=(A^2-A^1) = Portion of movement takingplace b/w acetabular component & acetabulum **(Outer bearing)**

Angle (B^3-A^3) = Portion of movement occurringb/w the head & acetabular component **(Inner bearing)**

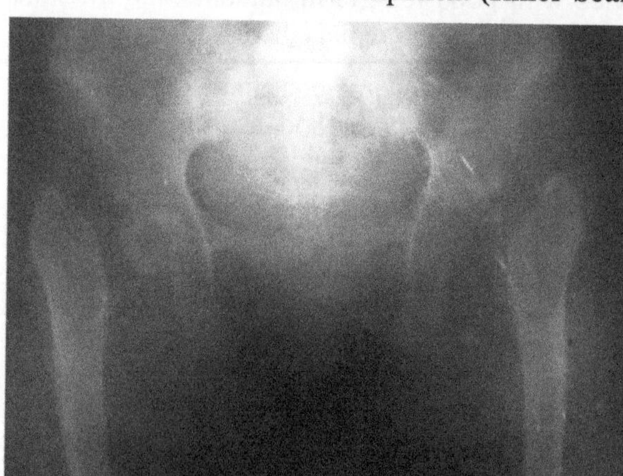

Case of B/L Osteomalacia with neck resorption

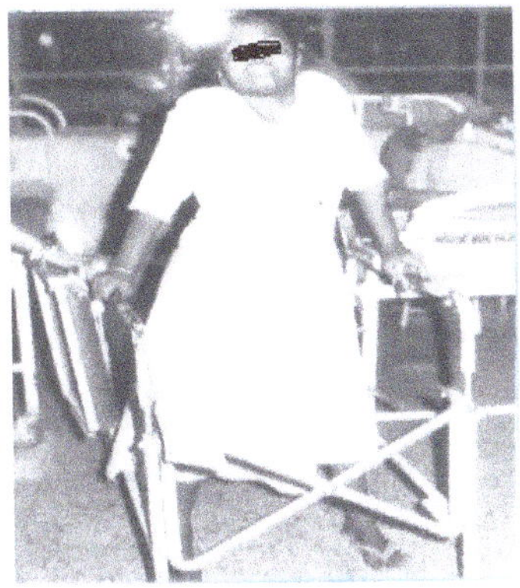

Pre OP Clinical Photograph of the same patient

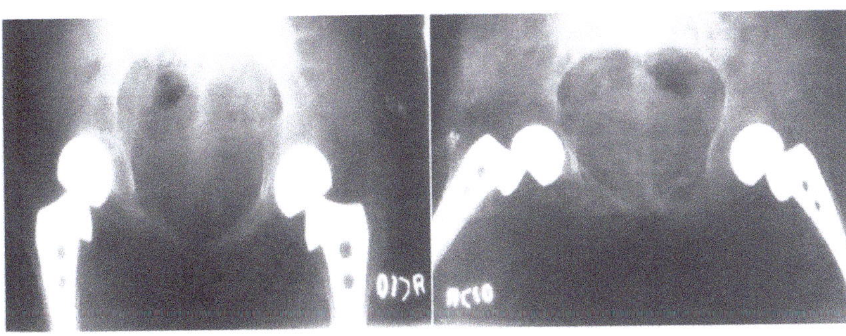

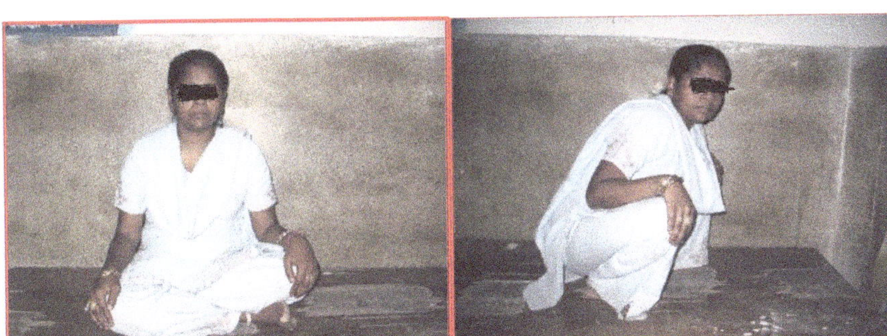

12 yrs post op of same osteomalacia patient; almost no impairment with preserved inner bearing movement.

What we found about inner bearing movement while using the BHU bipolar prosthesis at our institute has been summarised in the tables below.

Follow up duration	**Mean B^2 (degrees)**	**Mean A^2 (degrees)**	**Mean B^2-A^2(Degrees)**	**MeanB^2-A^2 (percentage)**
1.5 months	26.12	6.01	20.11	77.01
6 months	26.01	6.07	19.94	76.68
12 months	28.33	7.31	21.02	74.22
24 months	26.28	7.84	18.44	70.16
36 months	25.42	8.30	17.12	67.35
48 months	23.67	8.67	15.00	63.41
60 months	22.34	9.10	13.24	59.26
72 months	20.73	8.97	11.76	56.73
84 months	20.05	9.03	11.02	55.01
96 months	18.96	8.79	10.17	53.66
108 months	18.52	9.09	9.43	50.92
120 months	18.35	9.52	8.83	48.15

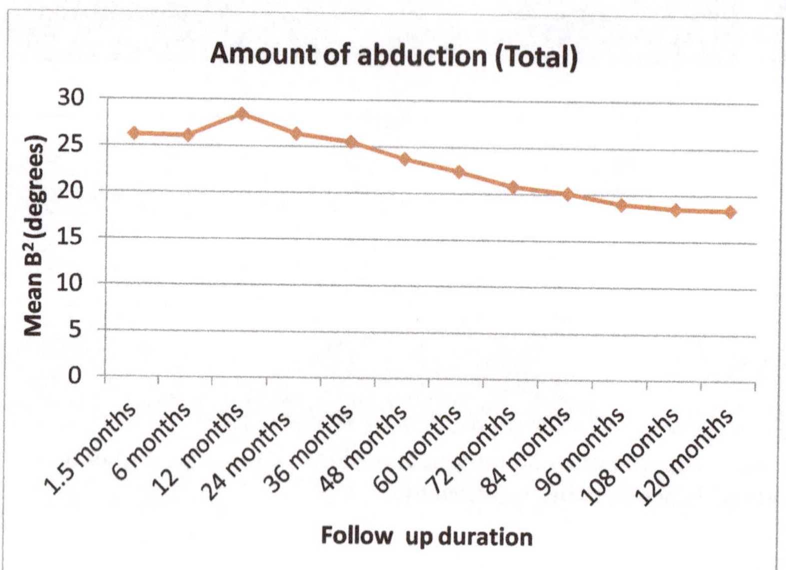

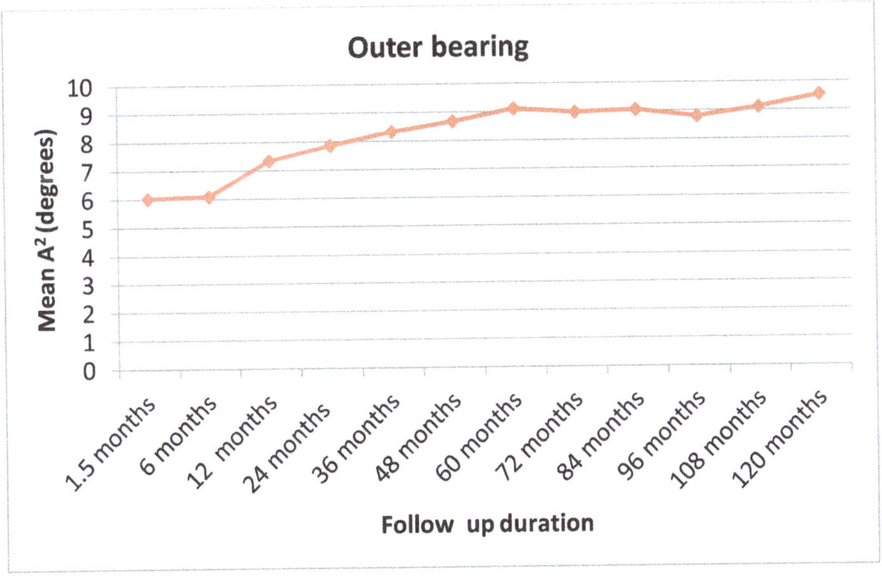
Outer bearing
Mean A² (degrees)
10
9
8
7
6
5
4
3
2
1
0
1.5 months
6 months
12 months
24 months
36 months
48 months
60 months
72 months
84 months
96 months
108 months
120 months
Follow up duration

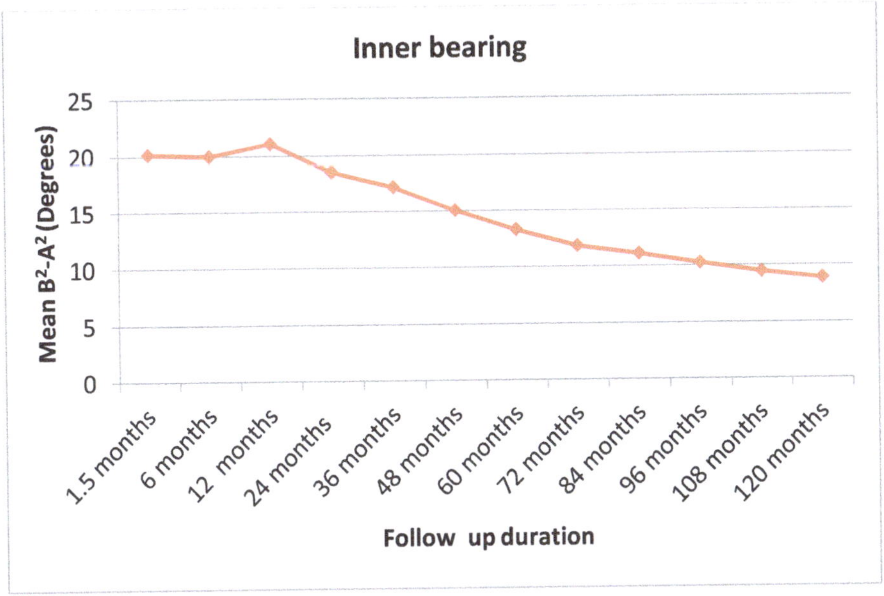
Inner bearing
Mean B²-A² (Degrees)
25
20
15
10
5
0
1.5 months
6 months
12 months
24 months
36 months
48 months
60 months
72 months
84 months
96 months
108 months
120 months
Follow up duration

Inner bearing movement analysis for arthritic hip

Follow up duration	Mean B^2 (degrees)	Mean A^2 (degrees)	Mean B^2-A^2(Degrees)	MeanB^2-A^2 (percentage)
1.5 months	26.28	14,16	12.12	46.12
6 months	24.22	13.02	11.20	46.28
12 months	23.67	13.50	10.17	43.00
24 months	21.11	12.04	9.07	41.30
36 months	19.42	12.00	7.42	38.21
48 months	18.12	11.49	6.63	36.60
60 months	17.32	11.36	5.96	34.42
72 months	16.18	10.87	5.31	32.86
84 months	15.58	10.73	4.85	31.15
96 months	15.12	10.53	4.59	30.40
108month	15.01	10.63	4.38	29.22
120 months	15.11	10.60	4.51	29.86

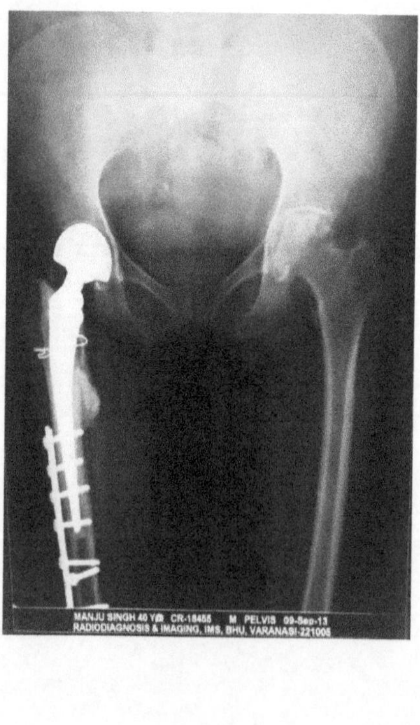

A 40 Years Old Female

History of Hip riplacement Rt Hip with Modular cemented Bipolar 7 yrs prior to presentation to us and plating was performed 2 yrs after first surgery for some trauma. Now presenting with AVN left hip.

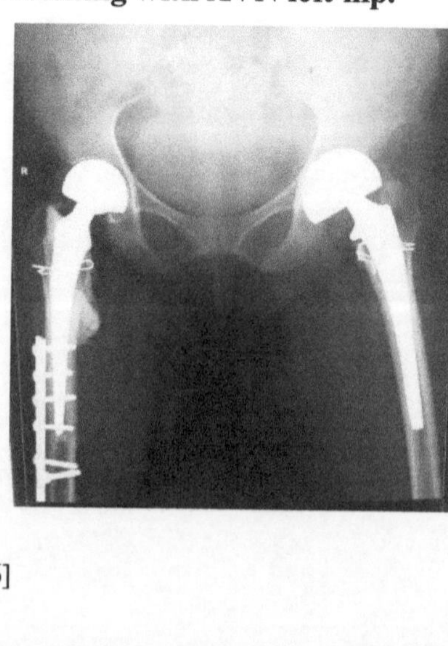

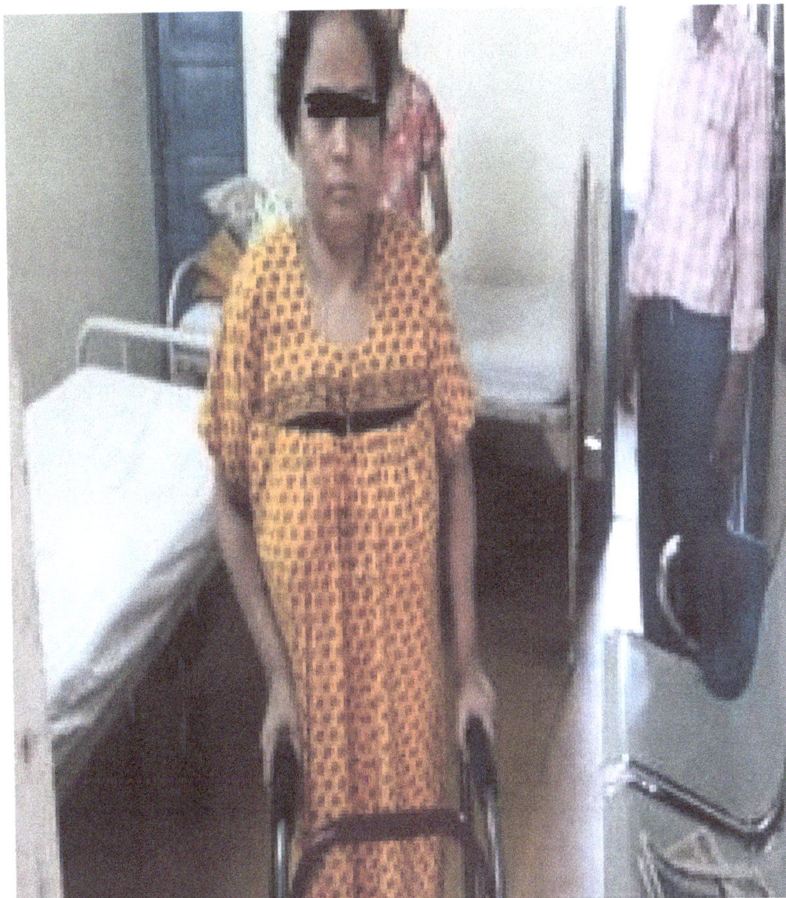

Left Hip Bipolar Arthroplasty (BHU Hip) after reeming the acetabulum up to 52mm & 52mm head was used without cementing the stem because the canal was very narrow. Mild fracture in the calcar was managed with circlage wiring.

Rationale for reaming being to accommodate a larger head hence thicker HMWPE along with 22 mm inner head, greatly increasing the longevity of prosthesis.

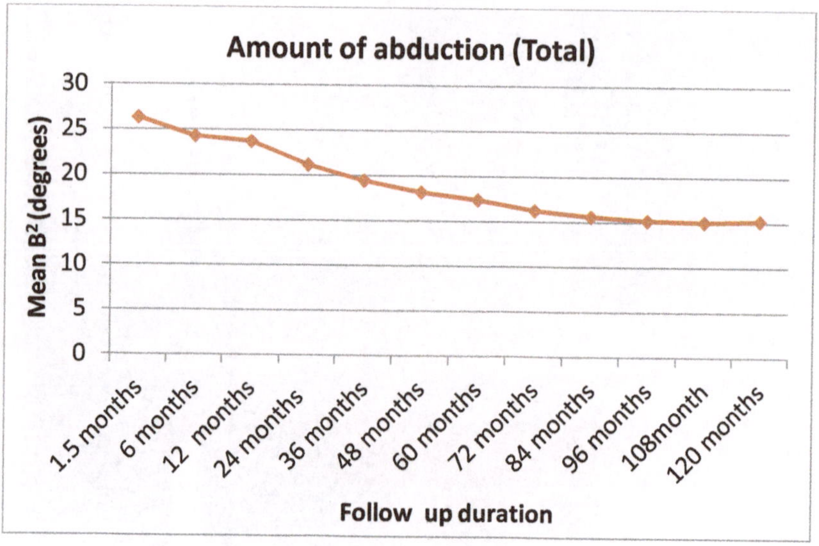
Amount of abduction (Total)
Mean B² (degrees)
30
25
20
15
10
5
0
1.5 months
6 months
12 months
24 months
36 months
48 months
60 months
72 months
84 months
96 months
108month
120 months
Follow up duration

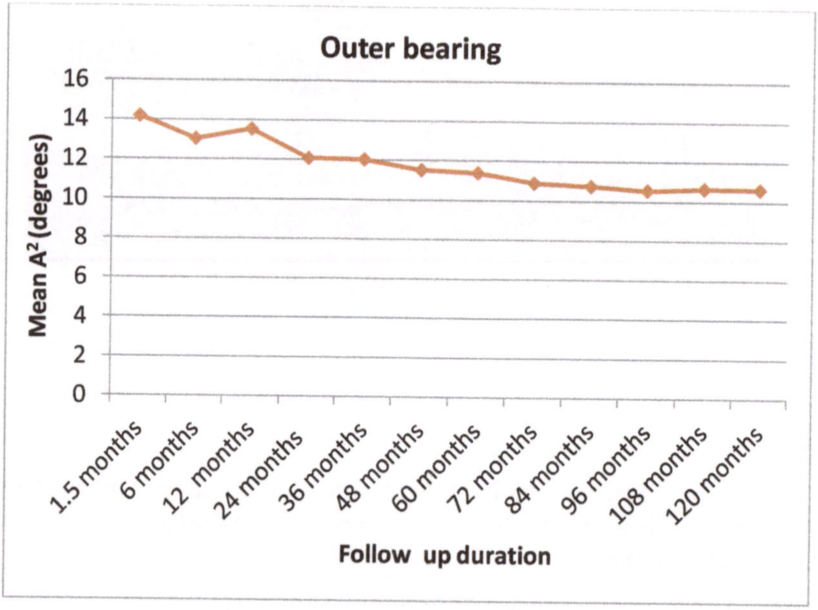
Outer bearing
Mean A² (degrees)
16
14
12
10
8
6
4
2
0
1.5 months
6 months
12 months
24 months
36 months
48 months
60 months
72 months
84 months
96 months
108 months
120 months
Follow up duration

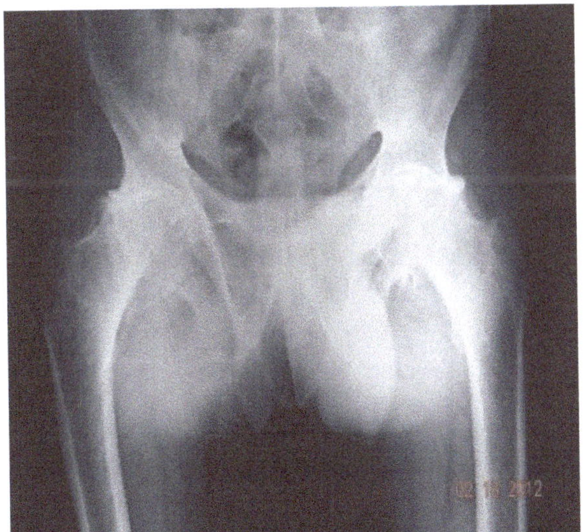

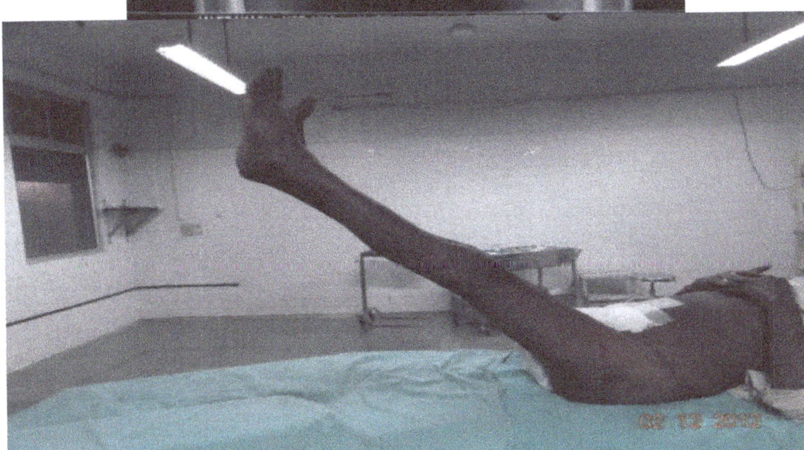

40 YEARS OLD MALE,ANKYLOSING SPONDILITIS WITH PAIN AND FIXED FLEXION DEFORMITY (45degree) OF BILATERAL HIP (L>R)

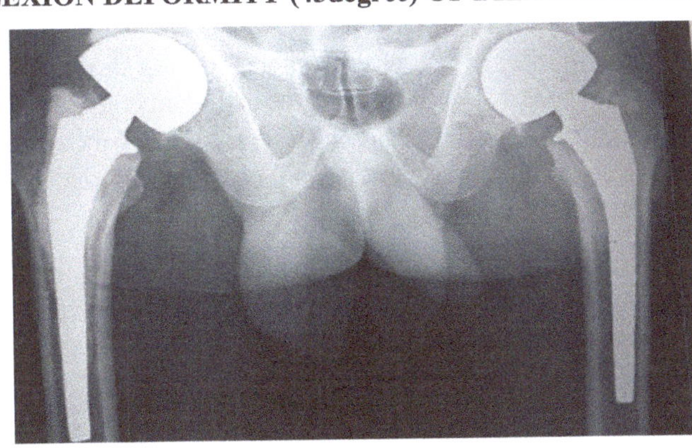

Bilateral Bipolar Hemi replacement arthroplasty was performed usingBHU Hip Device, cemented. Acetabular cavity was reamed in this case as well to have adequate socket and fitting of head.

8 yrs post op and patient s doing fine with pain free walking.

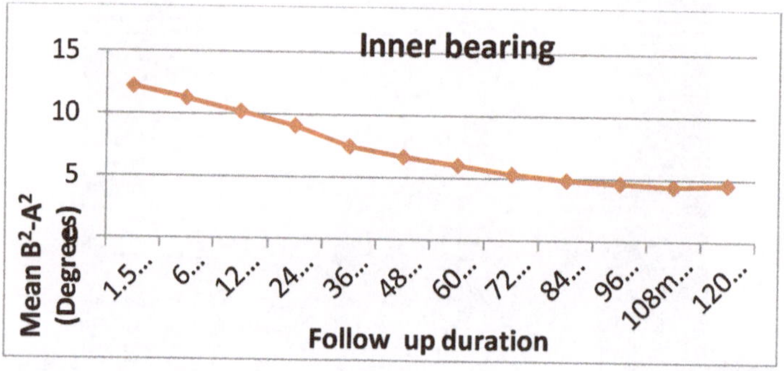

Inner bearing movement analysis for fracture neck of femur

Seen from the above observation it is clear that some movement was still present even after prolonged follow up.

As evident from the results the contribution of inner bearing movement to the total movement has been more in the cases where bipolar has been done for rough acetabulum as can be expected due to decreased outer bearing movement because of increased friction of coefficient between bone to metal interface.

Moreover there has been a gradual decrease in total movement of the joint as well as contribution from the inner bearing movement. The decrease in either of these movements has not been significant from one follow up to other but there has been a significant fall in movement compared from first follow up to last follow up.

There has been no significant decrease in inner bearing movement after five years of follow up and it might be due to some acetabular erosion that insinuates over that period of time leading to decreased movement at bone to metal interface and this phenomenon has been more evident in patients in whom the bipolar was done for fresh neck femur fracture.

At no point the total movement was exclusive, there was a persistent coexistence of motion between the two joints, and the inner bearing had fair contribution to the total movement which extended for quite a long post op period.

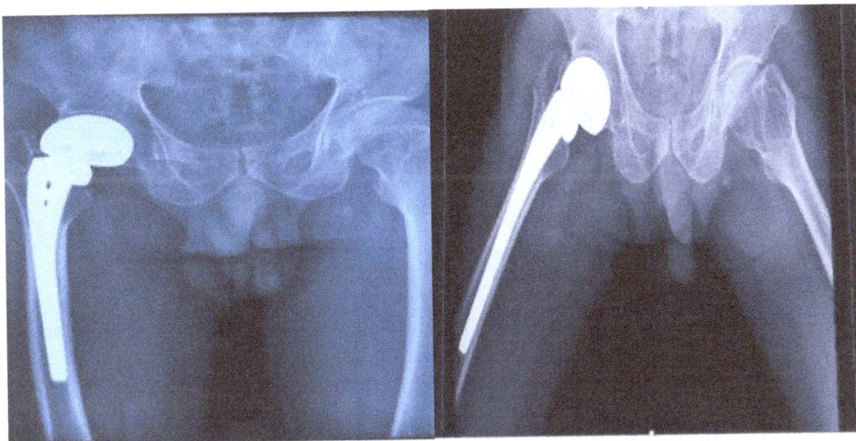

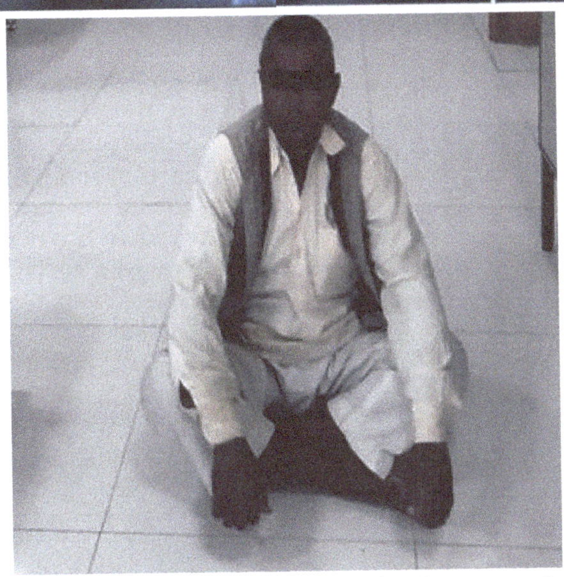

Post op 14th year follow up of bipolar hemireplacement done with BHU Bipolar for fracture neck of femur in a 60 yr old patient.

X-ray shows that not all the abduction is taking place at the outer surface that means some amount of inner bearing movement is still left(*contrary to findings of most of studies in past saying no inner bearing movement occurs only after few years*).

No acetabular erosion or protrusio and a pain free range of motion is also suggestive of same.

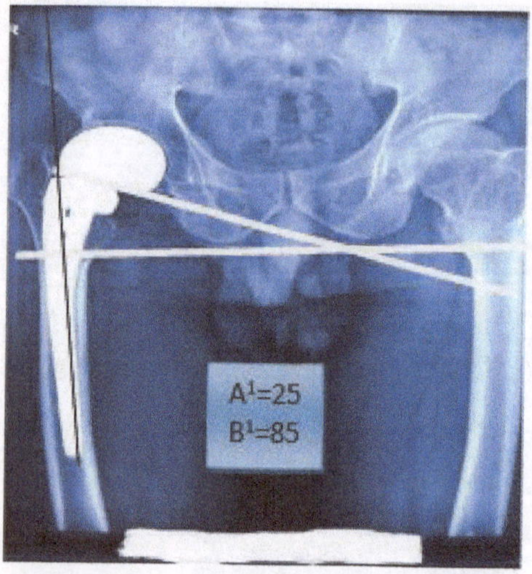

$A^3 = A^1 - A^1$ = motion between cup and acetabulum
$B^3 = B^1 - B^2$ = total abduction occurring
$B^3 - A^3$= motion at inner bearing 20*

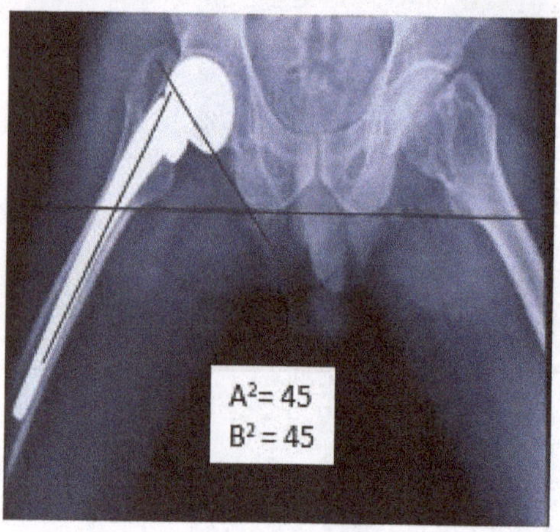

Clearly showing a movement of 20* at the inner bearing even after 12 yrs of post op, which is in contrast to what has been found in most of the studies in past which suggested that the bipolar device starts acting as unipolar within 1 yr of its application

Other than the justifiable use of prosthesis (like proper patient selection, proper approach and maintaining correct version and length.) there are several prosthesis related factors (as mentioned in chapter of designer changes as well) like

- offset of eccentricity,
- quality of polyethylene,
- inner head size
- shape of neck etc.
- seating angle
- head size in 1mm increments

That decides the continued motion at inner bearing.

In 1984 S.W Krein and E.Y.S Chao in their study Biomechanics of bipolar hip endoprosthesis where they used various designs of prosthesis to analyse the performance, demonstrated the role and effect of design of prosthesis on the final outcome. Hence the contribution of the design of prosthesis to overall success of surgery cannot be neglected.

The year long journey of turning the idea to the reality has gone through mind to mechanical lab to cadavers before coming to existence. After going through various articles on bipolar prosthesis many of them suggesting that bipolar starts acting as unipolar in a short span duration and after studying various bipolar designs we started working on the possible short comings. As brought to notice earlier as well impingement of neck over the polyethylene liner in extremes of motion leads to polyethylene debris insinuating an inflammatory response leading to fibrosis and hence problem in inner bearing movement. Moreover most of the bipolar prosthesis was such that calcar was not preserved due to the seating angle leading to sinking and later failure of device. Keeping these and various other points in mind we teamed up with the Mechanical department of BHU IIT and with their collaboration first the design idea was penned down on paper.

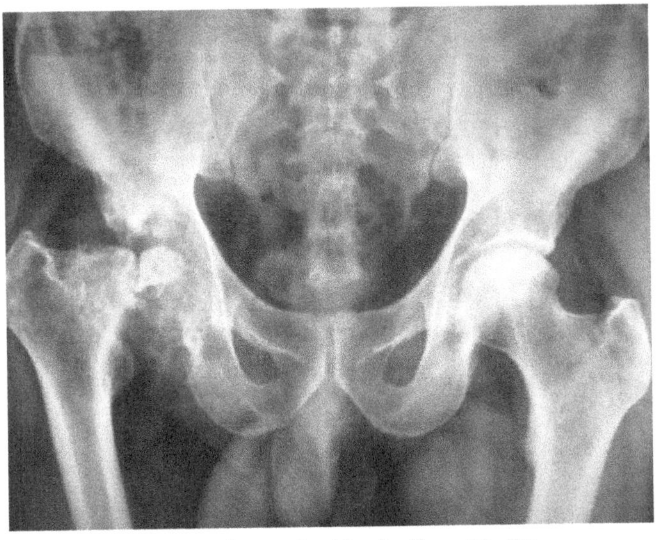

45yr/M Chronic Alcoholic with Rt. AVN Hip

On any given day with that kind of hip involvement on roentgenogramin a 45 yr old the usual and swift decision will be a Total Hip Replacement.

But with the flexibility in indications provided by the BHU bipolar we had the confidence to go ahead with Hemi replacement

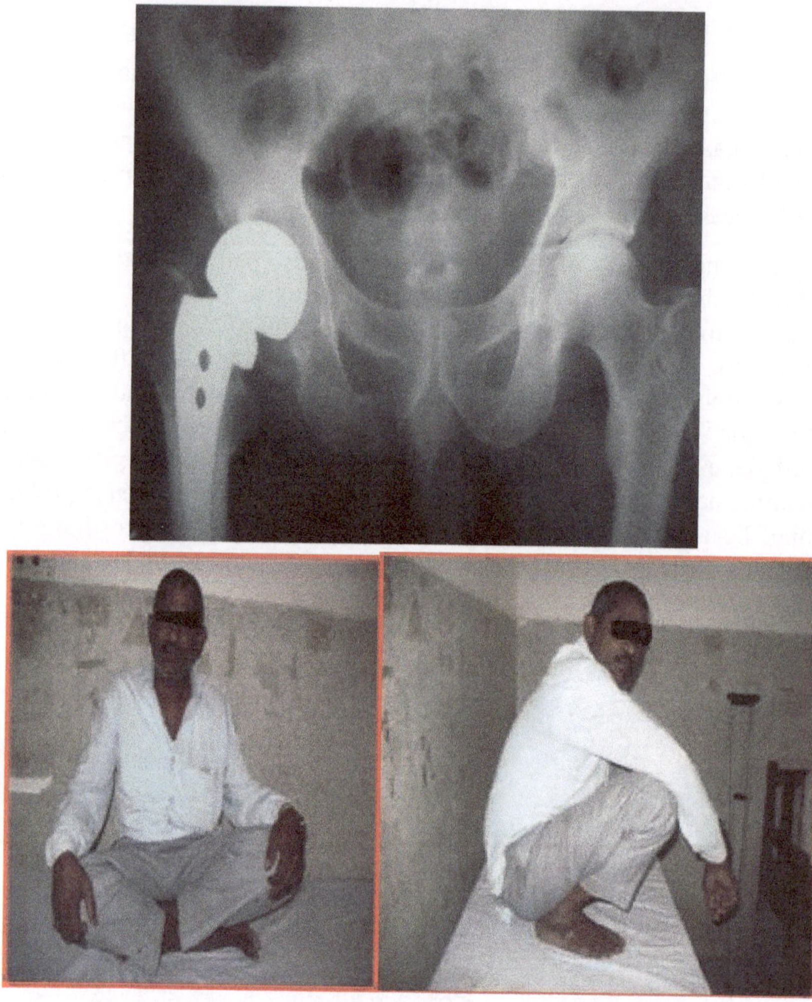

These are the x ray clinical pictures 14 yr post op of same patient.

No protrusio, calcar preserved, patient having pain free range of motion.

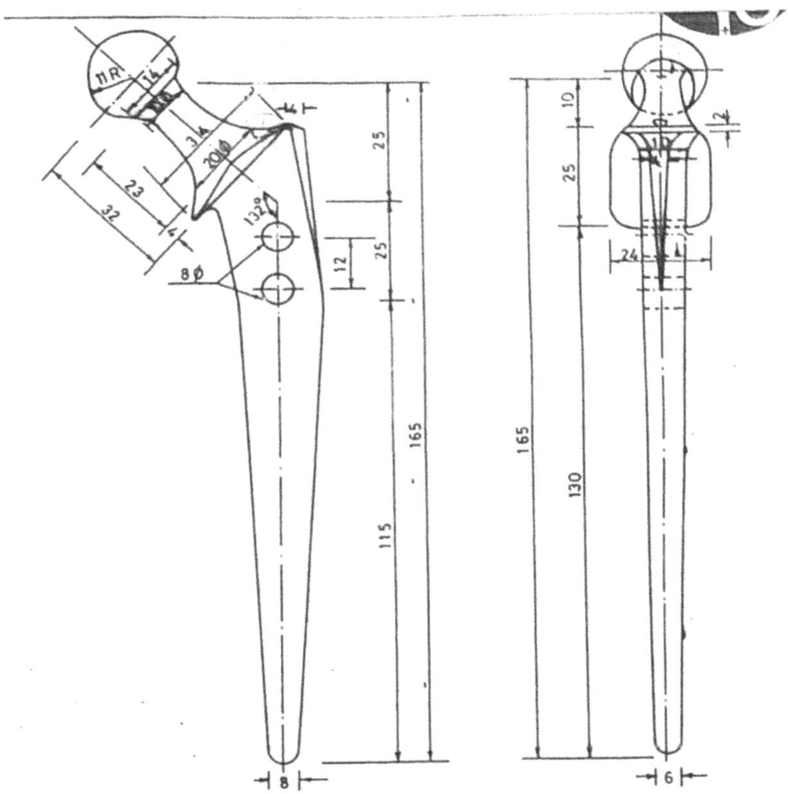

Wooden models were designed and refinements were made regarding adequate neck length for offset and stem thickness etcetera. Other designer considerations were also made as discussed in chapter of designer changes.

Aluminum prosthesis were made using these wooden models as template which were used for cadaveric studies to find out

(a) Best seating angle to preserve as much calcar as possible

(b) The adequate amount of calcar cut during surgery to have equal limb lengths post op

(c) The best possible version on insertion so that the prosthetic hip is as close as to normal hip as possible.

(d) Design of stem best in proportion to head size so that it snuggly fits in femoral canal, in metaphyseal area proximaly till its distal extent.

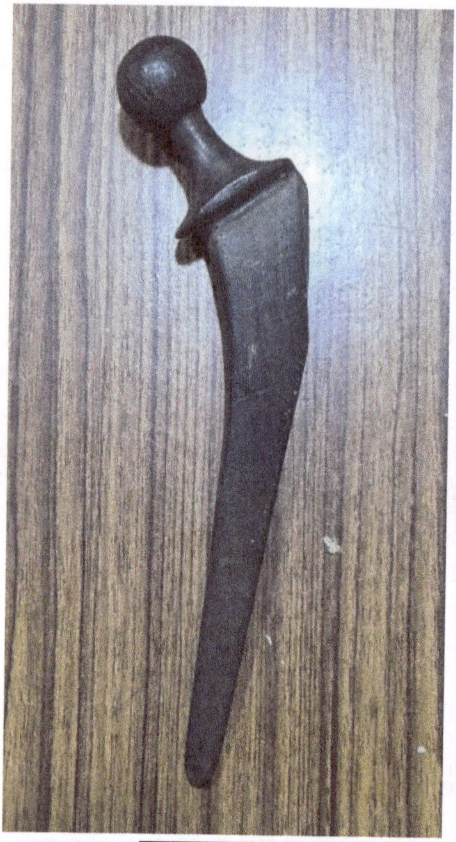 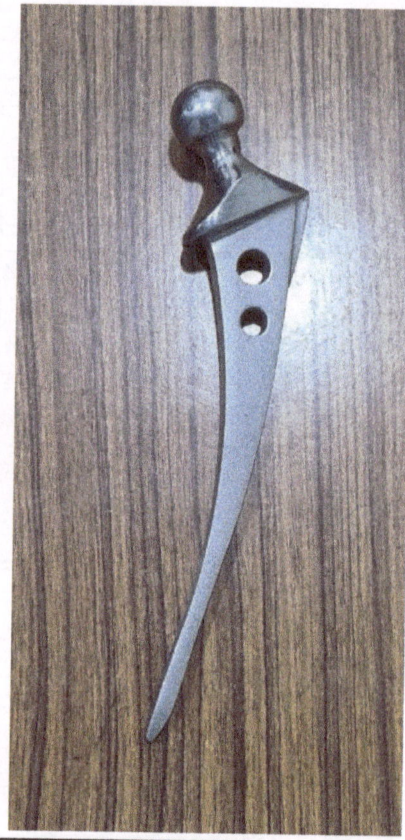

Wooden and aluminium models

In almost 99% of times we found that limb length are equal post operatively if we cut the calcar 1 cm above the lesser trochanter in Indian population, seating angle of prosthesis over the calcar was also modified on basis of cadaveric findings to preserve maximum possible calcar and least possible neck cup impingement. It was also found that if the posterior border of the prosthesis concedes with the anterior margin of lesser trochanter, version of prosthesis is close to the anatomical version. These technical details along with the designer refinements as discussed earlier made this prosthesis successful enough for us to try follow up for this long (10 years) which has been never done in past.

42 Year Old female (Rheumatoid Arthritis left hip)

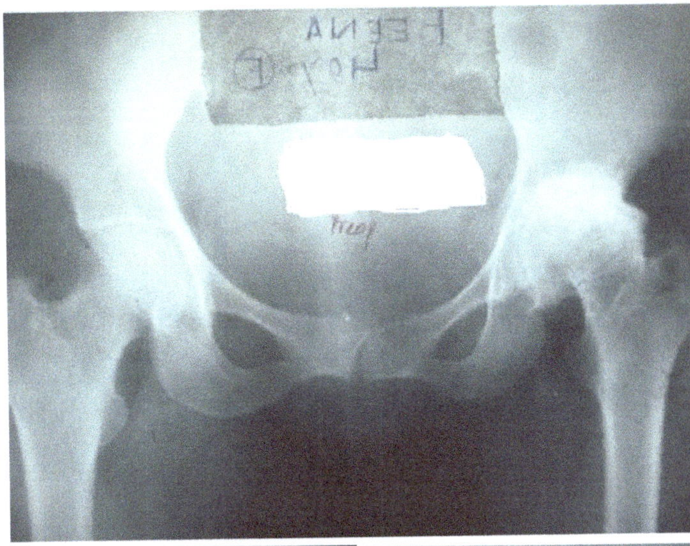

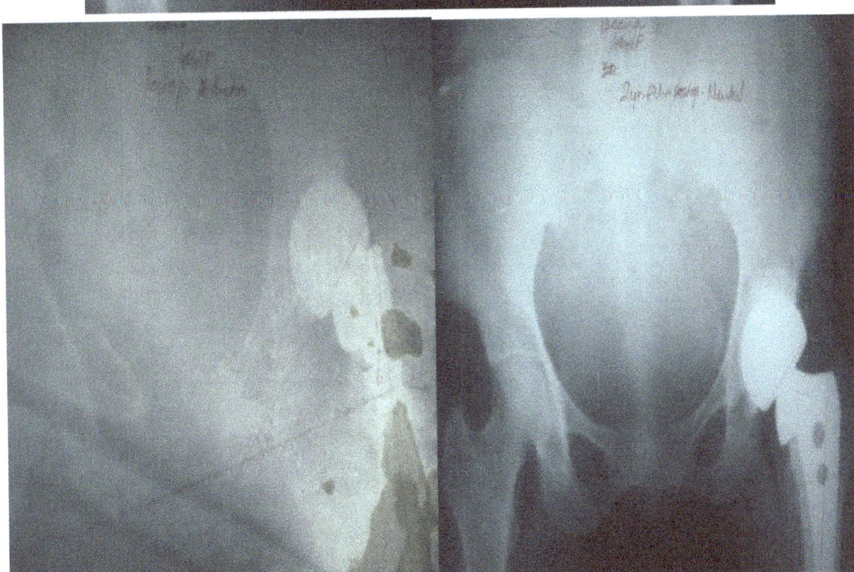

2 yr post op in abduction Neutral position

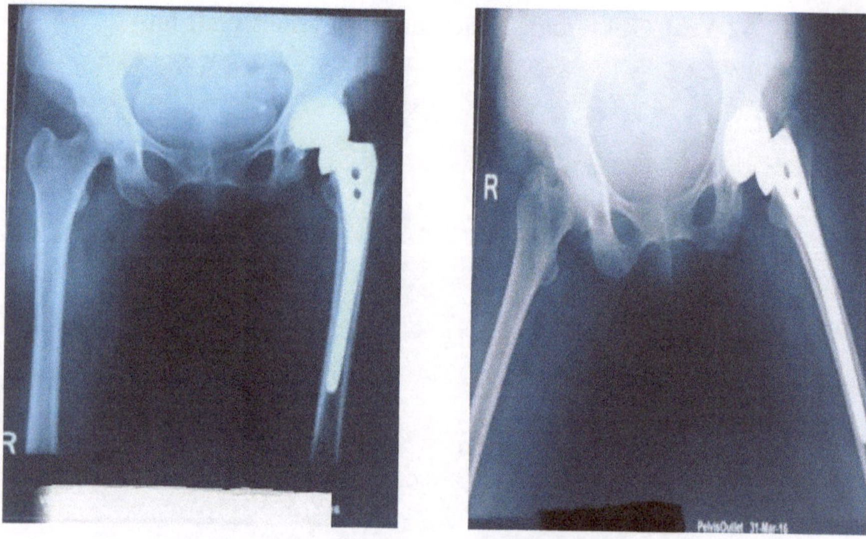

14 yr post op of same patient

Sitting cross leg and squatting in same patient

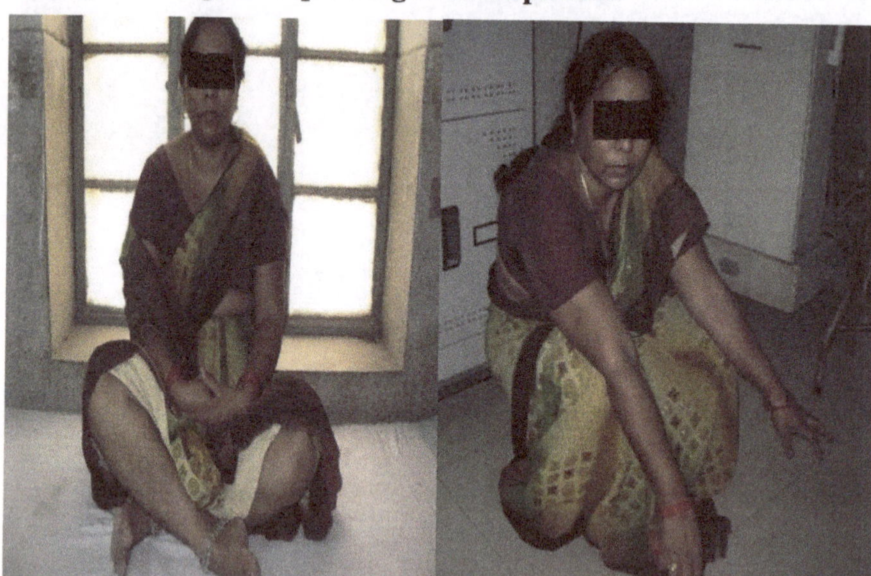

2yr post op and 14 yr post op x rays

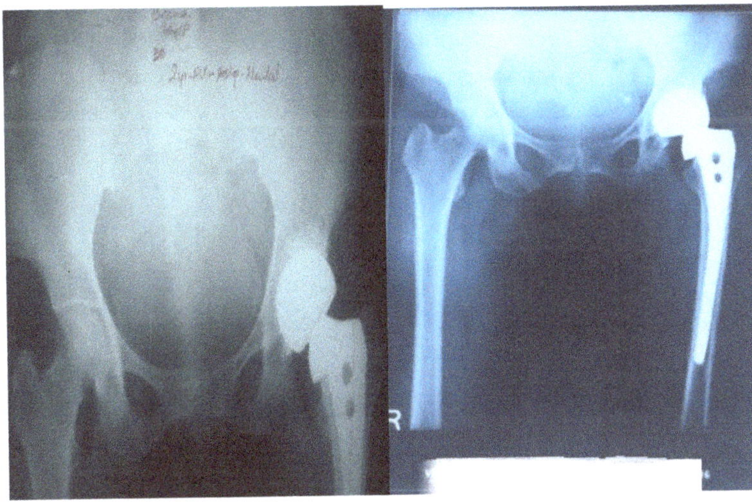

(a) (b)

A picture tells thousand story: no acetabular protrusion and sinking of prosthesis even after 14 yrs of post-op pain free walking, picture (a) 2yr post op & (b) 14 yrs post-op.

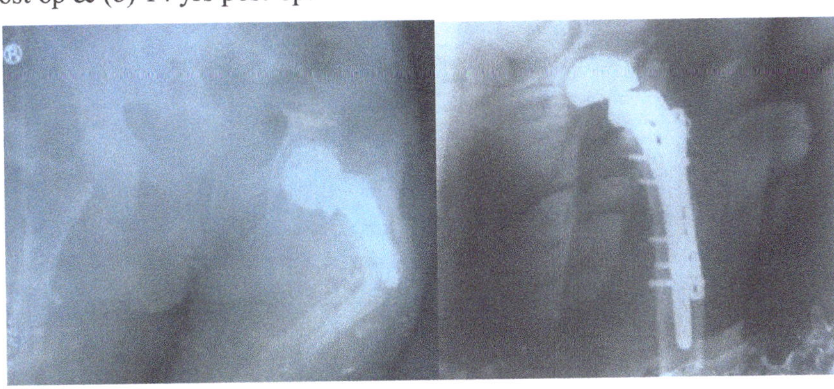

70 yr old female patient operated 10 yrs back came to us with broken Austinmoore is situ, BHU Hip device was applied along with plating. Patient happy to walk and carry out day to day activity on her own.

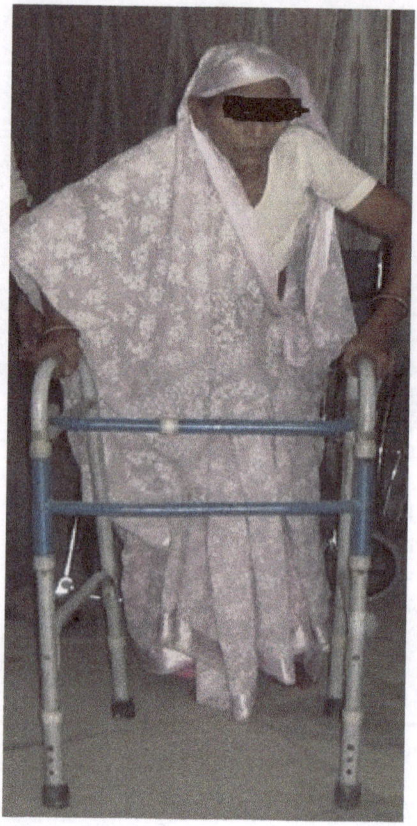

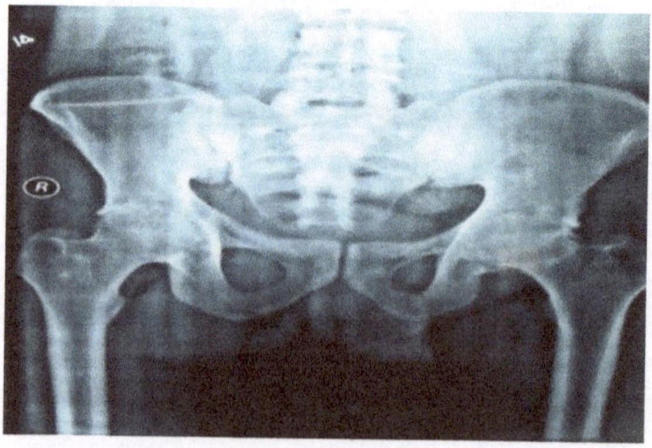

26 yr old male a case of ankylosing spondolytis with bilateral hip involvement. Financial constraints didn't allow us to do a total hip replacement so we went ahead and performed a staged both hip hemiarthroplasty with BHU bipolar.

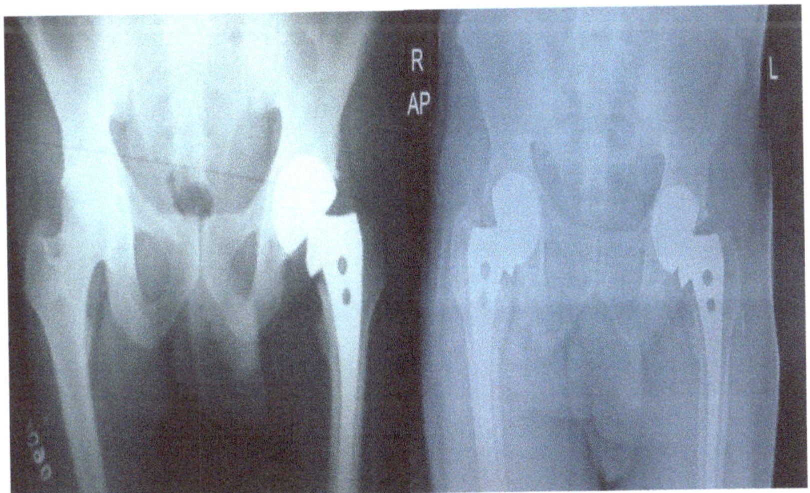

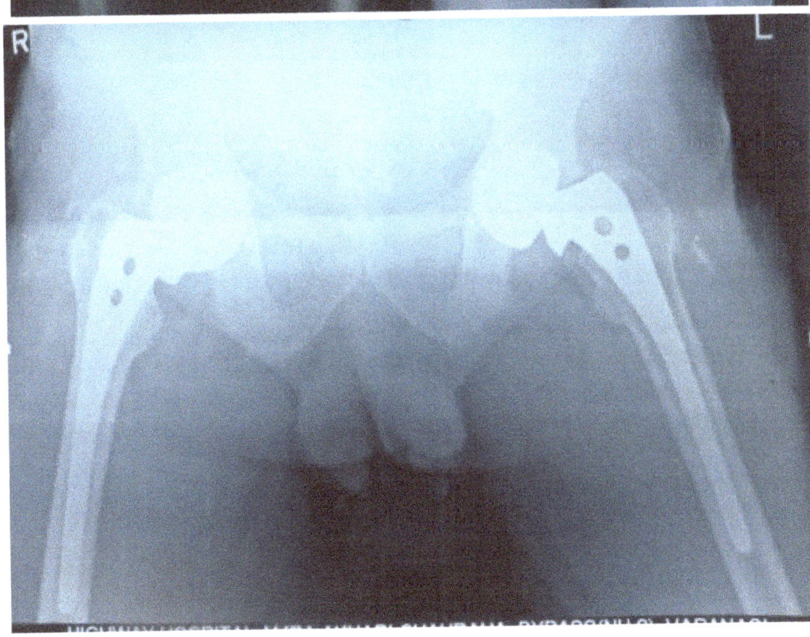

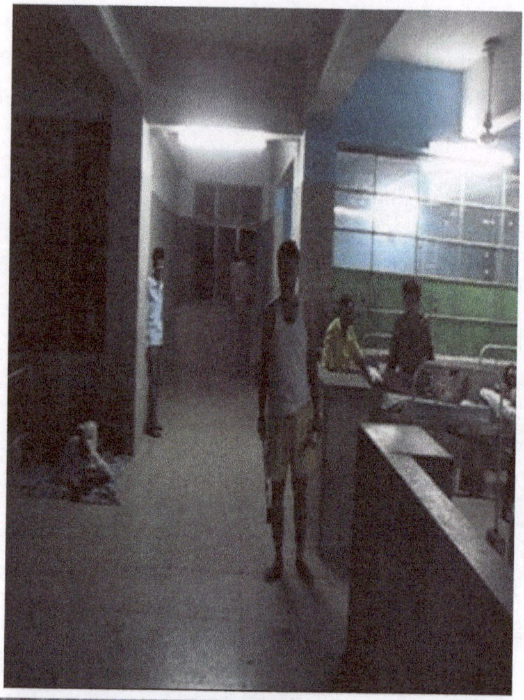

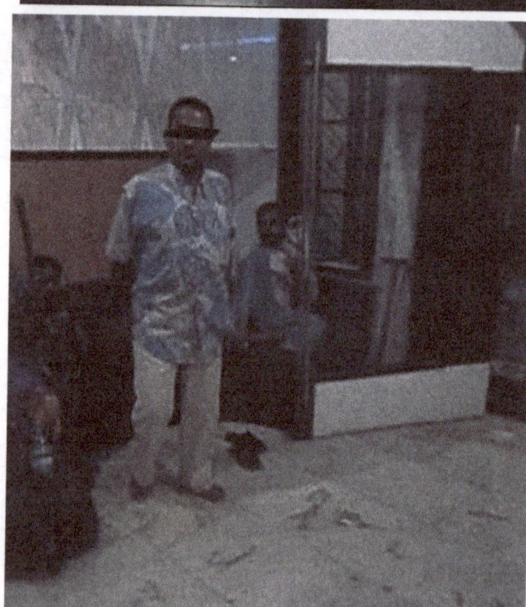

To everybody's surprise 15 yrs post op patient is able to walk pain free without any support, boosting the confidence on reliability of this prosthesis.

REFERENCES

1. GHM Verbrne. Femoral head prosthesis with built in joint: radiological study of movement of two component. JBJS 1983 Nov;65B(5).
2. . Drinker H, MurrayWR. The universal proximal femoral endoprosthesis :a short-term comparison with conventional arthroplasty. J Bone Joint Surg {Am}1979;61A:1167-74.
3. Lihong Fan, Xiaoqian Dang, and Kunzheng Wang Comparison between Bipolar Hemiarthroplasty and Total Hip Arthroplasty for Unstable Intertrochanteric Fractures in Elderly Osteoporotic Patients. PLoS One. 2012; 7(6): e39531. Published online 2012 Jun 22.
4. Feng Wang, Haifei Zhang, Zhiyu Zhang, Chengbin Ma & Ximin Feng Comparison of bipolar hemiarthroplasty and total hip arthroplasty for displaced femoral neck fractures in the healthy elderly: a meta-analysis. *BMC Musculoskeletal Disorders* volume 16, Article number: 229 (2015)
5. Jason BT Lim, Chia Liang Ang, and Hee Nee Pang. Acetabular Prosthetic Protrusio after Bipolar Hemi-Arthroplasty of the Hip: Case Report and Review of the literature. J Orthop Case Rep. 2016 Jul-Aug; 6(3): 28–31
6. Lestrange nr. the Bateman upf prosthesis: a 48 month experience. orthopedics 1979;2:373-377
7. Hedbeck CJ[1], Enocson A, Lapidus G, Blomfeldt R, Törnkvist H, Ponzer S, Tidermark J. Comparison of bipolar hemiarthroplasty with total hip arthroplasty for displaced femoral neck fractures: a concise four-year follow-up of a randomized trial. J Bone Joint Surg Am. 2011 Mar 2;93(5):445-50.
8. Soreide O, Molster A, Raugstad TS. Replacement with the Christiansen endoprosthesis in acute femoral neck fractures : a five year follow up study. Acta Orthop Scand 1980 ;51:137-44

FUTURE OF BIPOLAR PROSTHESIS

Polyehylene Lining

Polyethylene has been used successfully as the inner bearing surface in bipolar prosthesis as well as acetabular lining in case of total hip replacements. It was popularised by Sir John Charnley in his low friction arthroplasty hip. It has won its battle over other polymers like Teflon and Delrin. Ultra high molecular weight polyethylene became the most popular and standard material in THA since 1960s. The property that made it most suitable and favourable for use in replacement being It's semi crystalline nature which is constituted by a crystalline phase and an amorphous phase that allows some rearrangement of the crystals under mechanical stresses hence less brittle. The material had significantly large molecular weight meaning long polymer chains that are further reinforced by covalent molecular bridges also known as crosslinks.

However in early 90s long term survival ship of polyethylene came under scrutiny after incidences of osteolysis and aseptic loosening was brought to notice. Cement particles were first considered as causative agent and was so called the cement disease however this phenomena prevailed in uncemented designs as well.After significant research polyethylene debris particle was found to be the triggering mechanism. KJ Kim and HE Rubash In their study by histologic analysis revealed significantly large amount of polyethylene debris in bipolar replaced hip leading to membrane formation that produced great amount of prostaglandin due to inflammatory response leading to aseptic loosening and osteolysis. Verberne In his study back in 1980s mentioned presence of fibrous structure encircling the neck of the prosthesis making movements of inner bearing virtually impossible. On histologic examination it was found to be rich in foreign body giant cells which contained polyethylene debris.

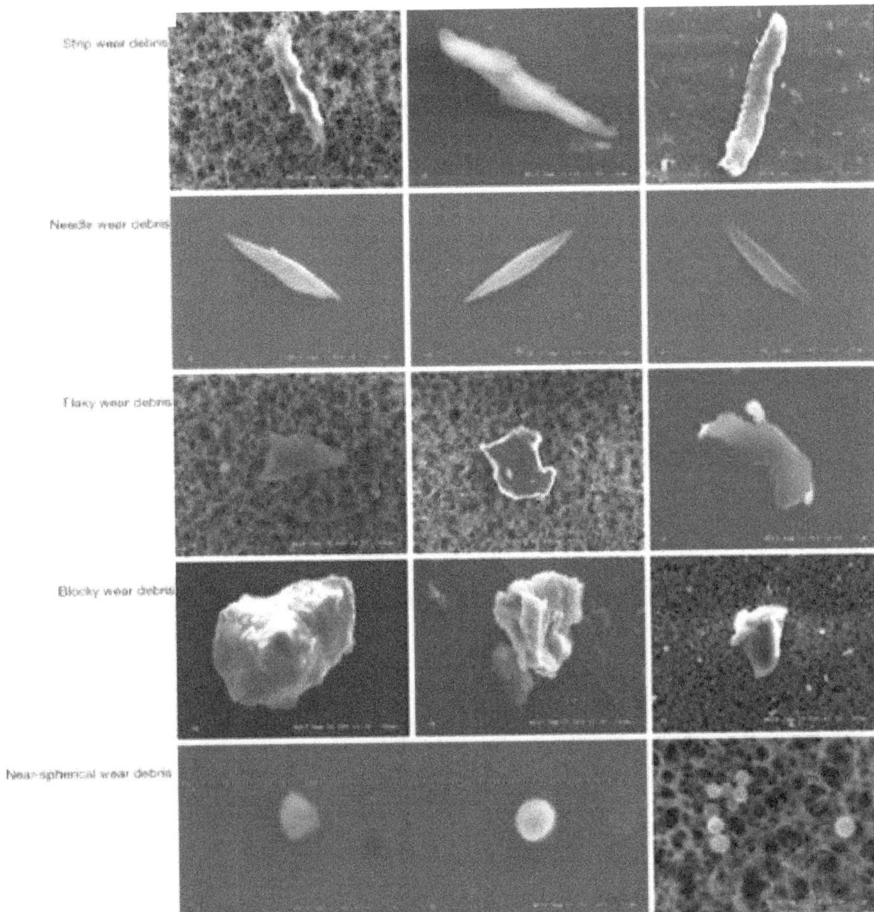

Extensive research was done to find out the cause of failure of polyethylene and to rectify it. It was found that there is a layer of subsurface white band in the components which has been kept on shelf for long moreover occasional fusion bond effects were also identified in the polyethylene components. It was later discovered that it is the oxidised polyethylene that constituted the subsurface white band and on mechanical analysis it was found to be comparatively brittle and prone for fractures. The gamma Irradiation has been the standard sterilization procedure for the polyethylene used for arthroplasty purpose which also promotes crossings between the large polymer chain. However this radiation in the presence of oxygen promoted the oxidation of the polyethylene leading to the subsurface brittle layer and it was more pronounced in the components kept on shelf for long. The first reaction to this problem was barrier packing to avoid oxygen permeability and perform gamma radiation sterilization in vacuum or in presence of inert gases and avoidance of implantation five years after manufacture and irradiation.

After long shelf life (5 years) of a gamma irradiated in air conventional polyethylene component, a subsurface white band is clearly detected.

But now the latest advancement is development of highly cross-linked polyethylene instead of ultra high molecular weight polyethylene which has got a notable increase in wear resistance it has been found in various studies that there has been a wear rate decrease ranging from 45% to 95% when highly cross-linked polyethylene was used instead of ultra high molecular weight however the rate of revision is yet to be established clinically. Highly cross-linked polyethylene definitely is a promising stuff for future use to reduce the polyethylene failure and to increase the longevity of the prosthesis.

Other antioxidant strategies are under development using different free radical scavengers such as vitamin E incorporation, HPAO (hindered phenol antioxidant) and many more.

Stem coating

Long-term success of the bipolar hemiarthroplasty is very much dependent upon the offset of processes and it's positioning into the femoral canal. Achieving the adequate offset depends upon the surgical skill of the operating personnel while maintenance of the achieved offset and stem positioning depends upon the quality of the bone. Leighton in his study in 2007 mentioned that the prosthesis offset is an important variable accounting for 99% of dislocation problems either anterior or the posterior approach used therefore he proposed that position of the femoral component and its primary stability has been the key to perform a successful stable hemiarthroplasty.

But this stability of the processes and the femoral canal becomes a challenge if the bone is of poor quality or the intramedullary canal is greater than 16.5 mm. This can lead to a risk of either proximal perioperative fracture or a late distal fracture secondary to the stress riser effect.

Answer to this problem for quite long in the past has been use of cemented fixation of the femoral stem in the femoral canal. However it has its own disadvantages, Parvizi in 2004 in his study 'thirty day mortality following hip arthroplasty for acute fracture' documented that mortality was more than doubled (3.5% versus 1.5%) when cement fixation was used. Many similar studies have agreed to the fact of increased rate of complications, when cement has been used for stem fixation especially in elderly population. Our findings at our institute were no different where operating and anaesthesia teams have to be on toes to avoid or identify development of any such complications when cement has been used.

Solution to this problem has been found in the form of coating of femoral stem to increase the bonding of prosthesis with bone especially for use in elderly osteoporotic bone with wide femoral canal. But this modality is still evolving in terms of material to be used for coating and the technique to apply that coating.

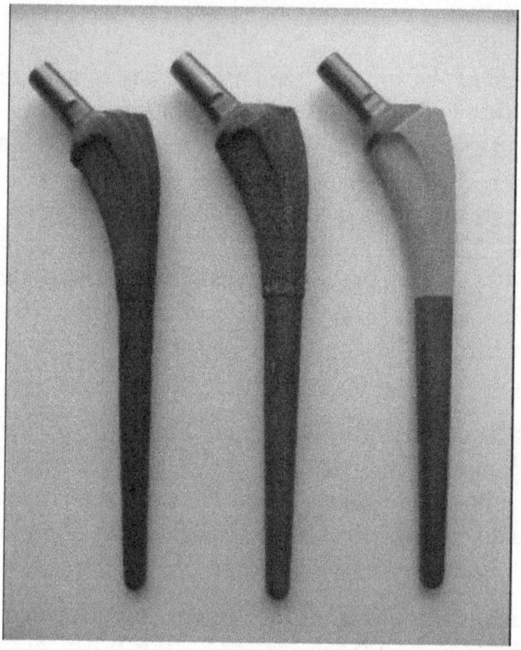

Schematically, the choice is based on three alternative principles:

•**material**: chrome-cobalt or titanium alloys;

•the principle of primary femoral fixation by adapting the bone to the prosthesis (straight, or "*European taper*"), or adapting the prosthesis to the bone (so-called "anatomic" or "personalized" components);

•secondary fixation, either by limiting bone growth in certain specific proximal areas, or promoting bone growth over the largest surface possible for completely micro porous implants.

Advances in the available options for uncemented stem have improved the osteointegration of bone to prosthesis stem. Most of these advances are mainly focused on increasing the roughness and porosity of the stem. Various methods that allows to do so are

Grit Blasting - The gritblasting process textures the metal surface with a pressurized spray of aluminum oxide grit or stainless-steel shot and resultsin an irregular surface (between 3 and 8 μm in depth)

Hydroxyapatite augmentation - In an attempt to further augment stem fixation, a hydroxyapatite coating is being used on metal substrate , this further can be only in the proximal part or on whole of stem. Result in either case is not much different however the proposed concept for whole length coating being a reduced stresses raiser effect. Plasma spray method usually applied for hydroxyapatite coating.

Proximal porous coating- hypothesis was that a proximal porous coating on the stem would result in better fixation and bone-remodelling than would a grit-blasted stem of identical design. Pure titanium porous coating are usually applied which is followed by hydroxyapatite coating .

However studies like one done by YE-YEON WON showed that proximal porous coating is not of much added advantage clinically in terms of repeat surgery or complain of pain however it gave better radiological outcome in terms of osteointigration, but this modality is still under evaluation for a long term follow up comparison.

MODULARITY IN BIPOLAR - Leighton in his study propagated the use of modular bipolar in neck femur fracture mentioning he reason that. a large size modular head can be used similarly ideal neck and head size can be used to maintain adequate muscle tension around the hip joint for optimum functioning of hip joint that automatically increases the longevity of prosthesis, and of course the ease to convert to Total Hip Replacement. However in practical scenario for fracture neck of femur if hemiarthroplasty has to be done then a proper use of technique (as mentioned in chapter of surgical approaches) will help achieving the desired offset and version. This is because the lesser trochanter and enough of calcar is spared during most of neck femur fracture to guide us for proper offset and and version of stem to be kept while doing hemireplacement.

Regarding the ease to convert to Total Hip Replacement, on realistic grounds most of the times its not only the neck and head assembly that has to be changed rather whole of the prosthesis has to be replaced . this might be because of the fact that in this Indian subcontinent affordability is one big issue and thus the kind of hemireplcement prosthesis used does not support modularity well, moreover with enhanced survival of the newer bipolar designs with preserved inner bearing movement for more than a decade as the one used at our institute has ruled out the need of THR in future in most of the cases.

But after all that has been said above there is no doubt about the fact that if the modularity is introduced to this existing bipolar design it will broaden the spectrum of use of this design.

Note-Practically cutting one centimetre (one finger breadth) above lesser trochanter gives equal limb length and thus modularitiy is undesirable in most of the situation in intra capsular fracture neck femur.

We cannot deny the fact that the scientifically introduced designer changes (refer to chapter of designer changes) that already exist in this design are also future based changes making it class apart prosthesis from other existing national or international prosthesis, but the evolution

is a continuousongoing process and there is always a scope of improvement even in the best.

Thus use of the latest kind of polyethylene with minimal wear rate , an adequate uncemented stem design and plus -minus introduction of modularity in this design in coming future can drastically enhance the longevity of this prosthesis and will make it a Future prosthesis.

References

1. Charnley J. Arthroplasty of the hip. A new operation. Lancet 1961;1(7187): 1129-32.
2. Medel FJ, Garcia-Alvarez F, Gomez-Barrena E, Puertolas JA.Microstructure changes of extruded ultra high molecular weightpolyethylene after gamma irradiation and shelf-aging. PolymerDegrad Stab 2005; 88(3): 435-43.
3. Gomez-Barrena E, Li S, Furman BS, Masri BA, Wright TM,Salvati EA. Role of polyethylene oxidation and consolidationdefects in cup performance. Clin Orthop Relat Res 1998; 352: 105-17.
4. Kurtz SM, Rimnac CM, Hozack WJ, *et al. In vivo* degradation ofpolyethylene liners after gamma sterilization in air. J Bone JointSurg Am 2005; 87A(4): 815-23.
5. Digas G, Karrholm J, Thanner J, Herberts P. 5-year experience ofhighly cross-linked polyethylene in cemented and uncementedsockets: Two randomized studies using radiostereometric analysis.Acta Orthop 2007; 78(6): 746-54.
6. Enrique Gómez-Barrena, Francisco Medel , José Antonio Puértolas. Polyethylene Oxidation in Total Hip Arthroplasty: Evolution and NewAdvances. *The Open Orthopaedics Journal,* 2009, *3,* 115-120
7. YE-YEON WON, MD, LAWRENCE D. DORR, MD, AND ZHINIAN WAN, MD. Comparison of Proximal Porous-Coated and Grit-Blasted Surfacesof Hydroxyapatite-Coated Stems. JBJS.ORGVOLUME 86-A · NUMBER 1 · JANUARY 2004
8. McCutchen JW, Collier JP, Mayor MB. Osseointegration of titanium implantsin total hip arthroplasty. *Clin Orthop.* 1990;261:114-25.
9. Engh CA, Hooten JP Jr, Zettl-Schaffer KF, Ghaffarpour M, McGovern TF,Macalino GE, Zicat BA. Porous-coated total hip replacement. *Clin Orthop.*1994;298:89-96.

10. Engh CA, Massin P, Suthers KE. Roentgenographic assessment of the biologicfixation of porous-surfaced femoral components. *Clin Orthop.* 1990;257:107-28. Erratum in: *Clin Orthop.* 1992;284:310-2.

11. Min B, Longjohn DB, Dorr LD, Wan Z. Radiographic comparison of diaphysealgrit blasted with smooth surface stems by matched pair analysis. *ClinOrthop.* 2000;381:156-67.

12. Dorr LD, Wan Z, Song M, Ranawat A. Bilateral total hip arthroplasty comparinghydroxyapatite coating to porous-coated fixation. *J Arthroplasty.*1998;13:729-36.

13. Rothman RH, Hozack WJ, Ranawat A, Moriarty L. Hydroxyapatite-coatedfemoral stems. A matched-pair analysis of coated and uncoated implants.*J Bone Joint Surg Am.* 1996;78:319-24.

Readers can revive following Papers published,

1-Journal of Trauma Management &
Outcomes

The BHU bicentric bipolar prosthesis in fracture neck femur in active elderly

Anil K Rai, Rakesh Agarwal*, Saurabh Singh and Ratnav Ratan
Address: Department of Orthopaedics, Institute of Medical Sciences, Banaras Hindu University, Varanasi-221005, India
Email: Anil K Rai - drakrai56@gmail.com; Rakesh Agarwal* - rakesh12280@gmail.com; Saurabh Singh - drsaurabhsinh@gmai.com; Ratnav Ratan - ratnav_ratan@yahoo.co.in

Published: 25 September 2008
Journal of Trauma Management & Outcomes 2008, 2:7 doi:10.1186/1752-2897-2-7
Received: 28 May 2008
Accepted: 25 September 2008
This article is available from:
http://www.traumamanagement.org/content/2/1/7

2-BICENTRIC BIPOLAR PROSTHESIS IN NON-TRAUMATIC HIP PATHOLOGIES: MAXIMUM 10 YEARS FOLLOW UP

Jha SC , Rai AK , Shakya P
DOI:http://dx.doi.org/10.3126/bjhs.v2i3.18934
* Corresponding Author
Dr. Subash Chandra Jha
Assistant Professor Department of Orthopedics Birat Medical College and Teaching Hospital
Tankisinwari, Biratnagar, Nepal
E-mail : subash.jha@gmalil.com

3-Bicentric bipolar hip prosthesis: A radiological study of movement at the interprosthetic joint

Anil Kumar Rai, Saurabh Singh, Vinay Kumaraswamy, GN Khare, Vinit Yadav, Rakesh Agarwal1
Department of Orthopaedics, Institute of Medical Sciences, Banaras Hindu University, Varanasi, 1
Ramkrishna Mission Hospital, Ranchi, India
Address for correspondence: Dr. Anil Kumar Rai,
C-209, Kamdhenu Apartment, Lanka, Varanasi - 221 005, India.
E-mail: anilrai56@gmail.com
DOI: 10.4103/0019-5413.87120

4-Journal of Clinical Orthopaedics and Trauma

Corresponding author. Department of Orthopedics Institute of Medical Sciences, BHU, 221005, India.
E-mail address: drsanjay.pgi@gmail.com (S. Yadav).
Contents lists available at ScienceDirect Journal of Clinical Orthopaedics and Trauma
journal homepage: www.elsevier.com/locate/jcot
https://doi.org/10.1016/j.jcot.2020.11.014

Note-Readers are requested to go throw the paper by Ramesh Bhandari which is an eye opening for the treatment options for inracapsular fracture neck of femur.

Open Access Protocol

BMJ Open

Hip fracture evaluation with alternatives of total hip arthroplasty versus hemiarthroplasty (HEALTH): protocol for a multicentre randomised trial

Mohit Bhandari,[1] P J Devereaux,[2] Thomas A Einhorn,[3] Lehana Thabane,[4] Emil H Schemitsch,[5] Kenneth J Koval,[6] Frede Frihagen,[7] Rudolf W Poolman,[8] Kevin Tetsworth,[9] Ernesto Guerra-Farfán,[10] Kim Madden,[11] Sheila Sprague,[12] Gordon Guyatt,[4] HEALTH Investigators

To cite: Bhandari M, Devereaux PJ, Einhorn TA, *et al*. Hip fracture evaluation with alternatives of total hip arthroplasty versus hemiarthroplasty (HEALTH): protocol for a multicentre randomised trial. *BMJ Open* 2015;5:e006263. doi:10.1136/bmjopen-2014-006263

▸ Prepublication history for this paper is available online. To view these files please visit the journal online (http://dx.doi.org/10.1136/bmjopen-2014-006263).

Received 13 August 2014
Revised 25 November 2014
Accepted 11 December 2014

For numbered affiliations see end of article.

Correspondence to
Dr Mohit Bhandari;
bhandam@mcmaster.ca

ABSTRACT

Introduction: Hip fractures are a leading cause of mortality and disability worldwide, and the number of hip fractures is expected to rise to over 6 million per year by 2050. The optimal approach for the surgical management of displaced femoral neck fractures remains unknown. Current evidence suggests the use of arthroplasty; however, there is lack of evidence regarding whether patients with displaced femoral neck fractures experience better outcomes with total hip arthroplasty (THA) or hemiarthroplasty (HA). The HEALTH trial compares outcomes following THA versus HA in patients 50 years of age or older with displaced femoral neck fractures.

Methods and analysis: HEALTH is a multicentre, randomised controlled trial where 1434 patients, 50 years of age or older, with displaced femoral neck fractures from international sites are randomised to receive either THA or HA. Exclusion criteria include associated major injuries of the lower extremity, hip infection(s) and a history of frank dementia. The primary outcome is unplanned secondary procedures and the secondary outcomes include functional outcomes, patient quality of life, mortality and hip-related complications—both within 2 years of the initial surgery. We are using minimisation to ensure balance between intervention groups for the following factors: age, prefracture living, prefracture functional status, American Society for Anesthesiologists (ASA) Class and centre number. Data analysts and the HEALTH Steering Committee are blinded to the surgical allocation throughout the trial. Outcome analysis will be performed using a χ^2 test (or Fisher's exact test) and Cox proportional hazards modelling estimate. All results will be presented with 95% CIs.

Ethics and dissemination: The HEALTH trial has received local and McMaster University Research Ethics Board (REB) approval (REB#: 06-151).

Results: Outcomes from the primary manuscript will be disseminated through publications in academic journals and presentations at relevant orthopaedic conferences. We will communicate trial results to all participating sites. Participating sites will communicate results with patients who have indicated an interest in knowing the results.

Trial registration number: The HEALTH trial is registered with clinicaltrials.gov (NCT00556842).

Strengths and limitations of this study

- This study has a large sample size of 1434 patients in order to detect small but important differences in outcomes.
- We are utilising an expertise-based randomised controlled trial design to help to eliminate differential performance and differential outcome assessments, and to reduce crossovers and ethical concerns associated with randomisation.
- The study has stringent methodological safeguards against bias including: use of a centralised randomisation system; blinding data analysts and the Steering Committee; standardisation and documentation; use of strategies to limit loss to follow-up; and adjudication of trial events by an independent Central Adjudication Committee.
- Surgeons and patients cannot be blinded to the surgical arms, leaving the assessment of outcomes and decisions to reoperate vulnerable to bias.
- We do not allow family members and friends to answer questionnaires on behalf of cognitively impaired patients; so some secondary outcomes will only apply to patients who are not cognitively impaired.
- The 2-year follow-up limits the study to shorter term outcomes.

INTRODUCTION

The number of hip fractures globally is expected to rise to over 6 million by the year 2050.[1,2] Owing to projected ageing of the

Summary-

1-The innovative design thus provide following, benefit.

2-No need of modularity becouse of 1cm preservation of calcar gives equal limb length. In intracapsular fracture in the active elderly group.

3-Long term survival (Minimum 21 years 2023).

4-Provide sitting and squating a cultural need.

5-Broad range of movement due to trapezyl neck of the design.

6-Easy operatalibility.

7-Less blood loss and operative time.

8-Provides normal gate.

APPENDIX

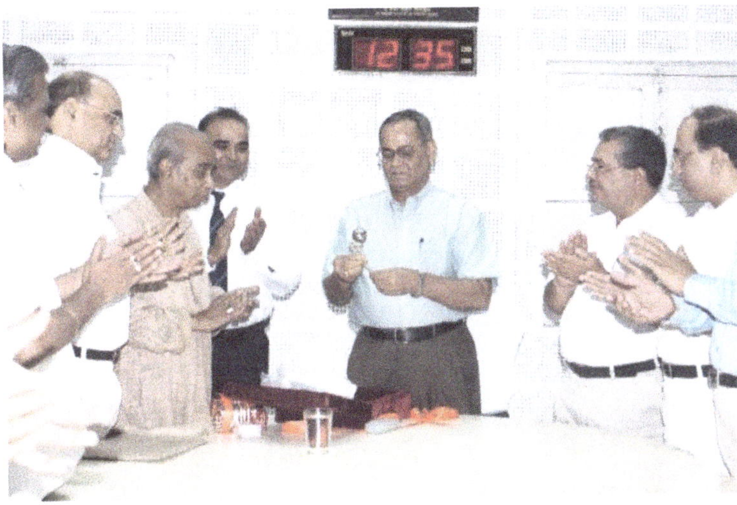

Inaugural Ceremony with EC Members & Vice Chancellor, BHU

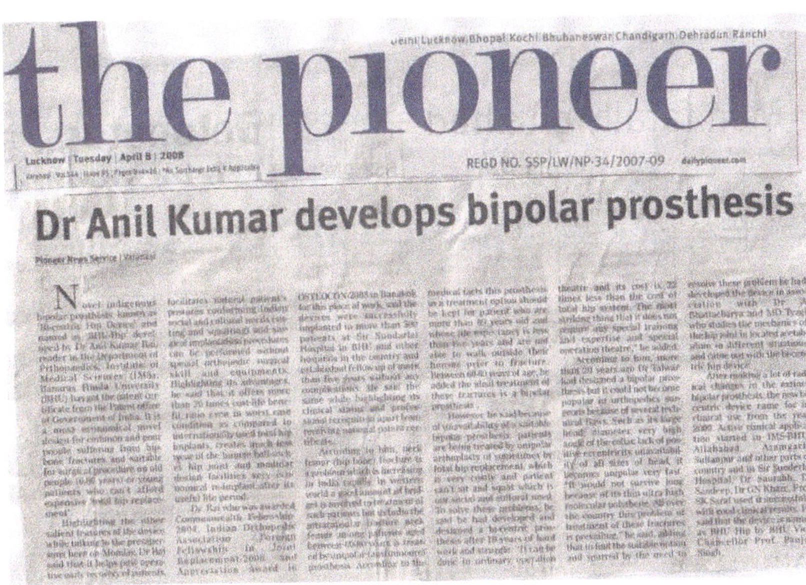

Delhi Lucknow Bhopal Kochi Bhubaneswar Chandigarh Dehradun Ranchi

the pioneer

Lucknow | Tuesday | April 8 | 2008

REGD NO. SSP/LW/NP-34/2007-09

Dr Anil Kumar develops bipolar prosthesis

Pioneer News Service | Varanasi

The Indian EXPRESS
www.expressindia.com

LUCKNOW | TUESDAY | APRIL 8 | 2008

BHU surgeon gets national patent for device to repair hip bone fracture

EXPRESS NEWS SERVICE
VARANASI, APRIL 7

ANIL Kumar Rai, a senior orthopedic surgeon from Banaras Hindu University (BHU), who developed and designed "Bi-Centric Hip Device" to offer flawless surgical cure to patients of Hip Bone fracture, has been awarded a national patent 216800(125/Del/1999) for the invention on March 24.

BHU Vice-Chancellor Panjab Singh named the device as 'BHU Hip Device' on Monday. Rai, a Reader at Department of orthopedics in the Institute of Medical Sciences (IMS-BHU), has worked at different hospitals in the UK before joining BHU. He developed the Hip Device after 10 years of hard work, along with Dr A Bhattacharya and M D Tyagi — from the Institute of Technology.

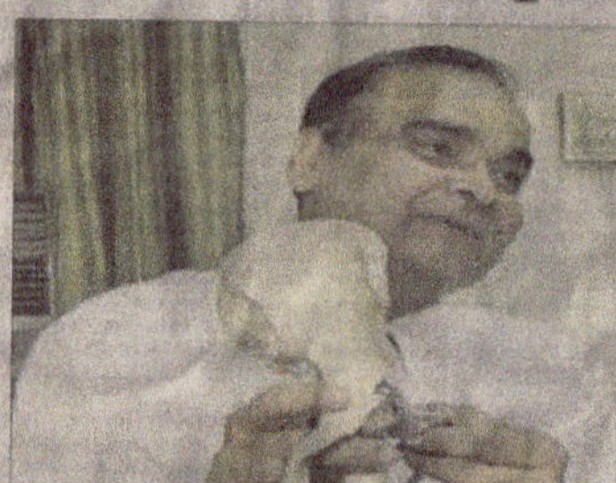

Dr Anil Kumar Rai at BHU on Monday.

"Patients of intra-capsular fracture neck femur (hip bone fracture), especially aged between 60 to 80 years, have either been treated by unipolar prosthesis or THR. In at least 50 per cent of such cases, these treatments do not deliver desired results," Rai told mediapersons on Monday. The purely indigenous device will be a boon for patients of hip bone (neck femur) fracture. According to sources, unipolar arthoplasty is a treatment best suited for those aged above 80 and has the life expectancy of less than two years.

THR on other hand, is an expensive surgery where the cost varies between Rs 1.5 to 1.8 lakh. "Even a successful THR cannot enable people to sit as well as squat with equal élan, which is the most common problem here," said Rai.

In such a scenario, the best possible surgical treatment for neck femur fracture is bipolar prosthesis. Owing to unavailability of suitable bipolar prosthesis, patients in India have either relied on unipolar option or THR, with the latter performed by surgeons specialized in THR at a well-equipped hospital.

Over two decades ago, one Dr Talwarkar had designed a bipolar prosthesis, but could not gain much popularity in the country due to technical flaws, such as large head, diameter, very high collar angle and lack of positive eccentricity. 'BHU Hip Device' is the most economical treatment of hip bone fractures which involves a cost of Rs 5,000 to Rs 10,000 (Rs 5,000 cost of device plus Rs 2,000 to Rs 5,000 as cost of surgery), which is 22 times less in terms of cost-life benefit even in worst case condition as compared to THR," Rai said. He added that the device besides being best suitable for patients between 60 and 80 years and young patients, who cannot afford expensive THR, also entails early post operative recovery, besides facilitating sitting and squatting.

Since 2000, the device has been successfully implanted in over 300 patients aged between 23 and 84 at BHU hospital and hospitals of Allahabad, Pratapgarh, Faizabad, Sultanpur, Azamgarh and Meerut and five year follow up of the patients suggests that the implanted device made from ultra-high molecular weight polythene can successfully function for more than 14 years. "The Molecular design of the device facilitates very economical (Rs 2,500) re-implant after its useful period is over", explained Rai, who now aspires to get a global patent for the device, being produced by a Gujarat based company.

Beginning of new era for Hip Hemireplacement

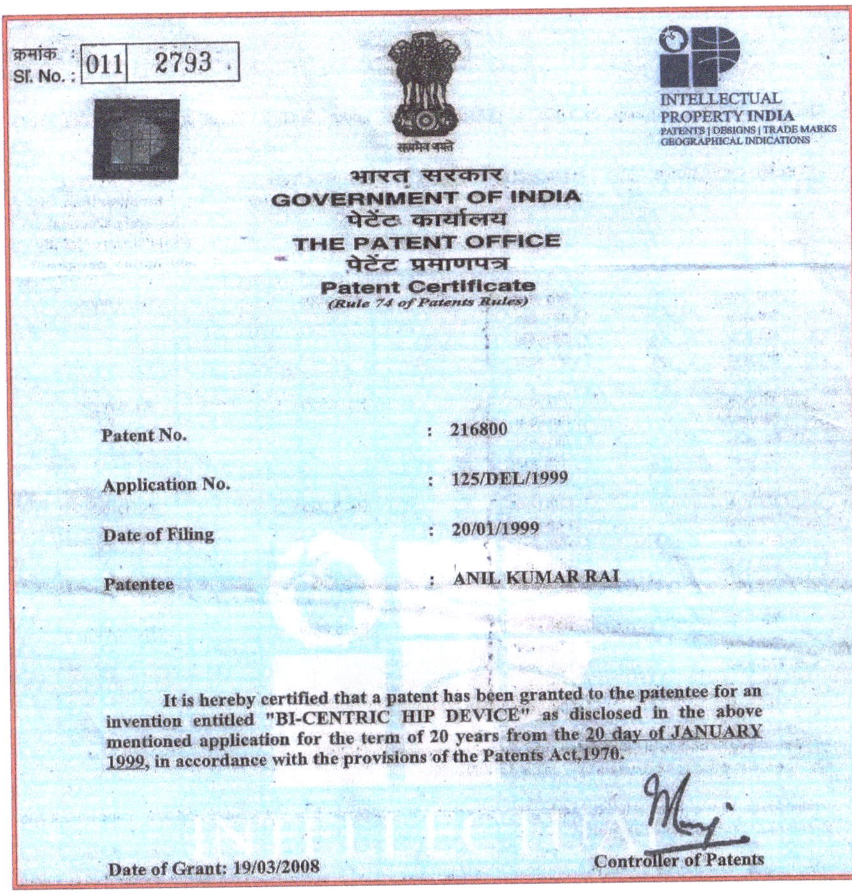

क्रमांक : 011 2793
Sl. No. :

सत्यमेव जयते

INTELLECTUAL
PROPERTY INDIA
PATENTS | DESIGNS | TRADE MARKS
GEOGRAPHICAL INDICATIONS

भारत सरकार
GOVERNMENT OF INDIA
पेटेंट कार्यालय
THE PATENT OFFICE
पेटेंट प्रमाणपत्र
Patent Certificate
(Rule 74 of Patents Rules)

Patent No.	: 216800
Application No.	: 125/DEL/1999
Date of Filing	: 20/01/1999
Patentee	: ANIL KUMAR RAI

It is hereby certified that a patent has been granted to the patentee for an invention entitled "BI-CENTRIC HIP DEVICE" as disclosed in the above mentioned application for the term of 20 years from the 20 day of JANUARY 1999, in accordance with the provisions of the Patents Act,1970.

Date of Grant: 19/03/2008

Controller of Patents

Patent certificate for the design of Prosthesis

Central Drugs Standard Control Organisation
Directorate General of Health Services
Ministry of Health & Family Welfare
(Medical devices and diagnostic division)

Food & Drugs Administration Bhawan,
Kotla Road, New Delhi-110002

No.: 29/MISC/3/2018-DC (223) **Date:** 8/6/2018

To,
Assistant Drugs Controller
1st Floor, Mata Anandamayee Hospital,
Shivala, Varanasi-221001,
Uttar Pradesh
E-mail ID: cdscoszvaranasi@gmail.com

Sub: Innovation total Hip replacement at BHU, Varanasi-Reg

Sir,

This has reference to the e-mail dated 13.04.2018 from Shri Anil Kumar Rai, Institute of Biomedical Sciences, Banaras Hindu University, Varanasi addressed to Hon'ble Prime Minister Shri Narendera Modiji on the subject cited above.(Copy enclosed)

Prof. Rai in his representation stated that their team alongwith Institute of Technology, BHU innovated "BHU HIP DEVICE". This devices costs only Rs. 6000/-and is a substitute to "total hip replacement" which costs Rs. 1.5 Lacs in majority of the indications which saves money for the common man. More than 10,000 patients have been treated at BHU and benefited. The device is patented and registered in their intellectual property act of India.

In this connection, you are asked to visit BHU immediately to understand the facts related to the matter of said orthopaedic implant and current status. The report along with all information may be forwarded to this office at your earliest.

The matter may be taken up on top priority.

Yours faithfully,

(Dr. V. G. Somani)
Joint Drugs Controller (I)

Copy to:
1. Shri Anil Kumar Rai, Department of Orthopaedics, Institute of Biomedical Sciences, Banaras Hindu University, Varanasi-221005 Email ID-anilrai56@gmail.com

Letter from Central Drugs Standard Control Organisation to Visit Institute for Prosthesis inspection.

Central Drugs Standard Control Organisation
Directorate General of Health Services
Ministry of Health & Family Welfare
(Medical devices and diagnostic division)

Food & Drugs Administration Bhawan
Kotla Road New Delhi-110002

No.: 29/MISC/3/2018-DC (223) Date: [illegible]

To,
Shri Anil Kumar Rai,
Department of Orthopaedics,
Institute of Biomedical Sciences,
Banaras Hindu University,
Varanasi-221005
Email ID-anilrai56@gmail.com

Sub: Innovation total Hip replacement at BHU, Varanasi-Reg

Sir

This has reference to your e-mail dated 13.04.2018 addressed to Hon'ble Prime Minister Shri Narendera Modiji on the subject cited above which is received by this office through proper channel

In this connection, it would be appropriate if you present your case for understanding the regulatory pathway approval before the CDSCO officials on 19 June 2018 at 12.15 PM at CDSCO HQ, FDA Bhawan Kotla Road, New Delhi. This is to assist you in understanding regulatory process i.e. how to make application for regulatory approvals, pre clinical, clinical trial requirements for early & proper regulatory approvals, etc

You are requested to provide information regarding regulatory status of the product in India along with pre clinical data of the product to this office for taking necessary action in the matter

Kindly acknowledge the receipt & confirm your arrival for presentation so that necessary arrangements can be made

Yours faithfully,

(Dr. V. G. Somani)
Joint Drugs Controller (I)

Copy to:
1. Assistant Drugs Controller, 1st Floor, Mata Anandamayee Hospital, Shivala Varanasi-221001, Uttar Pradesh

Letters of admiration for prosthesis design from Niti Ayog

डा. विनोद कुमार पॉल
सदस्य
Dr. Vinod K. Paul
MEMBER

सत्यमेव जयते

भारत सरकार
नीति आयोग, संसद मार्ग
नई दिल्ली-110 001
Government of India
NATIONAL INSTITUTION FOR TRANSFORMING INDIA
NITI Aayog, Parliament Street
New Delhi-110 001
Tele. : 23096809 Telefax : 23096810
E-mail : vinodk.paul@gov.in

June 14, 2019

Dear Professor Rai,

I enjoyed going through the materials of BHU Hip Device. This innovation is highly promising and gains attention and visibility.

Please do meet me on my next visit to BHU and demonstrate the project.

With regards,

Yours faithfully,

(Vinod K Paul)

Prof. Anil Kumar Rai
Head of Department
D/o Orthopedics
Institute of Medical Sciences
Banaras Hindu University
Varanasi

स्वच्छ भारत
एक कदम स्वच्छता की ओर

डॉ. विनोद कुमार पॉल
सदस्य
Dr. Vinod K. Paul
MEMBER

सत्यमेव जयते

भारत सरकार
नीति आयोग, संसद मार्ग
नई दिल्ली-110 001
Government of India
NATIONAL INSTITUTION FOR TRANSFORMING INDIA
NITI Aayog, Parliament Street
New Delhi-110 001
Tele. : 23096809 Telefax : 23096810
E-mail : vinodk.paul@gov.in

9th May, 2019

Dear Dr. Rai,

The Office of Hon'ble Minister for Health and Family Welfare has forwarded your letter of 19th February, 2019 addressed to the HFM. I am pleased to note that you have developed a bipolar prosthesis, namely, the BHU HIP Device.

I am sure this innovative product, developed and made in India, is of considerable potential. I would be delighted to know more about this product when I visit BHU in the near future. In the meanwhile, kindly let me know what we can do to promote this product in a scientific manner.

Warm regards,

Yours sincerely,

(Vinod K. Paul)

Prof. Anil Kumar Rai
Head of Department
D/o Orthopedics
IMS-BHU
Varanasi

स्वच्छ भारत
एक कदम स्वच्छता की ओर

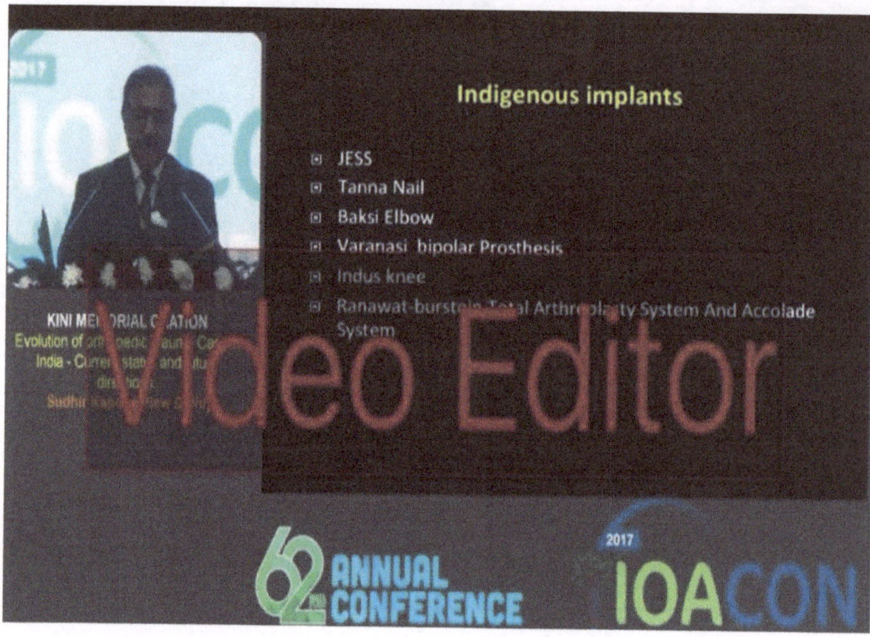

Acknowledging the prosthesis design as indigenous Implant list in KINI Memorial Oration IOACON 2017